LIVING WITH IT

LIVING WITH IT

WHY YOU DON'T HAVE TO BE HEALTHY TO BE HAPPY

SUZY SZASZ

PROMETHEUS BOOKS
BUFFALO • NEW YORK

Living With It: Why You Don't Have to be Healthy to be Happy

Copyright © 1991 by Suzy Szasz

All rights reserved. No part of this book may be reproduced in any manner whatsoever without written permission, except in the case of brief quotations embodied in critical articles and reviews. Inquiries should be addressed to Prometheus Books, 700 E. Amherst Street, Buffalo, New York 14215, 716-837-2475.

95 94 93 92   5 4 3 2

Library of Congress Cataloging-in-Publication Data

Szasz, Suzy.
   Living with it : why you don't have to be healthy to be happy / by Suzy Szasz.
     p.   cm.
   ISBN 0-87975-659-4
   1. Szasz, Suzy—Health. 2. Systemic lupus erythematosus—Patients—United States—Biography. I. Title.
RC924.5.L85S98   1991
362.1'9677—dc20   90-27045
                                                                                  CIP

Printed in the United States of America on acid-free paper

For my father

My father, in all his teaching, demanded of me not only the utmost that I could do, but much that I could by no possibility have done.
—John Stuart Mill

Preface

> I have never been anywhere but sick. In a sense sickness is a place, more instructive than a long trip to Europe, and it's always a place where there's no company, where nobody can follow.
> —Flannery O'Connor

I have been ill most of my life. There has never been any question in my mind about that fact. I knew I was sick long before I had an official diagnosis, Systemic Lupus Erythematosus—usually called "SLE" by physicians and simply "lupus" in everyday English. Lupus is an autoimmune disease, which means that the body produces antibodies against some of its own cells, resulting in damage to connective tissue in any part of the body (hence lupus is also called a "connective tissue disease"). Typically, the symptoms include fatigue, joint pains, low-grade fever, muscle aches, and general malaise. The disease is chronic and life-long, characterized, in some cases, by periods of near-complete remission, in others, by quiescent periods with occasional exacerbations of lupus activity, called "flares."

I never denied that I was ill. However, unlike the hypochondriac who wants to be accepted as a patient, I have always wanted to be accepted as a non-patient, a person whose primary identity is something other than being a patient. This story is about growing up ill, being ill, nearly dying twice but surviving, and trying, always, to be something more than a professional patient. Although this story is about me, I would not call it an autobiography. I am not an important enough person to write an autobiography. My aim is to make this the story of an experience, rather than of an individual. While the particular events in my story are unique, the lessons they teach about living with a chronic illness are, I believe, universal. Although I don't regard lupus as a stigma and am not writing under a pseudonym, out of respect for the privacy of others I have changed the names of places, other persons, and the details of some events that may embarrass others.

There are many accounts available today about the misfortune of being stricken by terrible diseases, written either by survivors or people close to them. Whatever the reasons for the emergence of this literary genre—ranging, perhaps, from intellectual curiosity to morbid exhibitionism-plus-voyeurism—the popularity of both fictionalized medicine and medicalized fiction is secure. Regardless of the disease discussed, most display one or more of the following features. The author is a well-known person, for example, Joseph Heller, *No Laughing Matter,* or Betty Rollins, *First You Cry.* A variation on such celebrity medical autobiographies offers the public accounts of "recoveries" from non-diseases, for example, *Darkness Visible: A Memoir of Madness* by William Styron, or *Now You Know* by Kitty Dukakis. The saga is sometimes told by someone other than the victim, who watched a loved-one struggle and die nobly, for example, John Gunther, in *Death Be Not Proud,* Gerda Lerner, in *A Death of One's Own,* or Philip Roth, in *Patrimony: A True Story.* In some cases, the subject is an *acute* disease that is cured or goes into complete remission: Guillain-Barre syndrome (again, Joseph Heller) or breast cancer (Betty Rollins). The author/survivor often attributes his success in conquering a supposedly dread disease to an unconventional intervention, for example, Norman Cousins, *Anatomy of an Illness as Perceived by the Patient.*

* * *

I hope to do something different, namely, to tell the tale of the life of an unknown young woman; to write it myself, in my own words; to explain what it is like to live with a chronic illness rather than have it go into remission or recover from an acute condition; to recount how I have learned to manage my illness working with doctors, not against them—how I have been helped by scientific treatments not quack cures; to discuss not only the medical details of my disease, but its financial aspects as well; and, finally, to describe what it is really like to live with lupus *without* remission—and yet have something to show for my life other than coping with an illness.

This book is based on my own recollection of events that I find relevant to my experience of living with lupus. The story is presented chronologically, but—except for the near-fatal flare I suffered in 1983, during which time I kept a journal—it is not based on a diary. While at times I attempt to speak as a fourteen- or a twenty-four-year-old, I wrote as a thirty-four-year-old reflecting on only those incidents that remain important to me. As a result, there are times where seemingly significant scenes lack detail, and others where the details may seem excessive. In recreating episodes from the last twenty years of my life, I have tried not to embellish or belittle them. Lastly, while I reveal a great deal of my personal life, I have deliberately kept some details private.

People like to read about other people's battles with terrible diseases (whether or not they recover), especially if they are rare illnesses unlikely to strike them. But as the likelihood of living out one's life with a debilitating chronic illness increases, the threat of such a calamity strikes increasingly closer to home. The lack of literature on living with a chronic illness may be due to one simple fact: The drama of day-to-day life with a chronic illness is, plainly, not very dramatic. Unlike an acute, life-threatening disease that one heroically overcomes or tragically succumbs to, chronic illness is unremitting, and, for the most part, uneventful. In a way, it is like life itself, unrelenting, often boring. That is why people like to dramatize their dilemmas with quack cures, ranging from religious adventures in the grottos of Lourdes to pseudo-medical adventures in the back alleys of Tijuana. Thanks to medical advances, more and more people are now living with diseases "under control" but not "cured." In addition, scientific progress has made many people view medicine as a mystical enterprise, capable of solving the world's problems. As people's expectations rise and are, inevitably, unfulfilled, they reject scientific medicine and embrace quackery. "It has not yet occurred to the layman," observed Alistair Cooke, "that doctors—like cab drivers, schoolmasters, politicians, and television repairmen—can be very good, good, indifferent, bad, or downright stupid."

The patient's proper role in living with a chronic illness is vastly different from his role in dealing with an acute disease. To be sure, in neither case should the patient be held responsible for his illness. No doubt that is why patients are typically described as "victims," who must "battle," "overcome," and "triumph" over their illnesses. None of these words accurately describes what the patient with a chronic illness must do. If such an individual sees himself as a victim, he is doomed. Why? Because acting the victim implies helplessness and passivity, in short, lack of control. Instead, the patient with a chronic illness must recognize that while he is not responsible for his disease, he is responsible, and must take responsibility, for its management. In a sense, this makes living with a chronic illness not very different from living without one: For everyone, healthy or sick, living competently requires assuming maximum responsibility for one's own life.

For me, having a chronic illness for most of my life made shouldering such responsibility, perhaps paradoxically, easier. I could use my illness and the necessity to take care of it as a guidepost for taking care of my life as a whole. At times, my illness narrowed the range of choices open to me, compared to those of my healthy friends. But it also encouraged me to take charge of my life early, instead of aimlessly going with the flow, a behavior so common in my generation. Also, I discovered that even during the worst episodes of my generally quiescent illness, when my options narrowed precipitously, I still had free will over my life. Some people may believe that only those of us who come close to death can fully appreciate the value of free will. I don't place the ill in such a special category: Anyone who aspires to live a responsible life, healthy or sick, must place autonomy high on his list of values.

Obviously, no two healthy people live their lives the same way, even if given the same opportunities. Similarly, no two sick people manage their illnesses exactly the same way, even if they have the same disease, the same doctors, and the same treatments available to them. In the end, each person must manage his life in a way that makes sense to him, for it is he who must live with its consequences.

As every biologist knows, we begin to die the minute we are born. Normally, it's a slow enough process. For me, the process has been accelerated. How much, no one knows for sure. So, while I have a progressive illness, the uncertainty of its prognosis makes me think more about living and less about dying. And more about living *well*. As I grew up, ill, I came to believe strongly that the purpose of life was not to live as long as medically possible (as if one could ever make sure of that), but to live as competently, contentedly, and with as much self-determination as possible.

Finally, I would like to acknowledge several people who have helped me with this book. My gratitude to my father, who read and re-read each and every draft of the manuscript, is implicit in these pages. In addition, special thanks go to John Badgley, who was spared reading all but the last revision, but managed nonetheless to be nearly as critical as my father. And I am indebted to Bob Basil, senior editor at Prometheus Books, for assigning Reg Gilbert to edit the final version. Reg's conscientiousness, competence, and devotion have been the realization of every fledgling author's dream.

March 23, 1991

One

> The doctor may also learn more about the illness from the way the patient tells the story than from the story itself.
> —James B. Herrick

It was Monday, February 21, 1983.

"Miss Szasz? I hope I'm not disturbing you. May I come in?"

Was the high fever, hitting 105 several times a day, every day, affecting my hearing, if not my brain? A person who has never been a patient in a modern American hospital may see nothing unusual in this introduction. I was called "Miss Szasz," rather than Susan. And the "visitor" acknowledged that he was an intruder and asked permission to speak with me.

I had been in the hospital longer than ever before in my twenty-seven years. The events of the previous eleven days were beginning to dim this remarkably fortunate fact. In the midst of what seemed to be an endless procession of doctors, nurses, and technicians, here stood yet another unfamiliar and unwanted face before me in my room. It was early evening, long after dinner and the regular hours of the doctors' hospital rounds.

Who was this tall man with a warm smile on his face and no white coat on his back? By now, I had seen the head of virtually every department in Lyman Memorial hospital. Perhaps he was just another of the many physicians affiliated with this private hospital (or with Mansfield General, the adjoining university teaching hospital) who had been told about this "interesting case" and wanted to see "it" for himself. In any event, his civilized approach aroused my curiosity. I sat up in bed, interested to hear more.

"Yes, of course. Come in."

* * *

Although I am no longer annoyed by hospital personnel addressing me by my first name, I cannot help being aware of how demeaning it can be. I am now in my mid-thirties, and at less than five feet tall, look younger. Many of the people I encounter in medical settings are close to my own age. Still, I have always noticed that in virtually all medical situations—in the waiting room of the X-ray department, in the clinical laboratory, in physical therapy—rarely does a physician or paraprofessional address a patient by his last name. It makes no difference whether the professional is older, younger, or the same age as the patient. Sex doesn't matter either. At the same time, rarely, if ever, have I heard a patient address a member of the medical community by his first name. While I dislike that practice just as much, if such reciprocity prevailed I could attribute the phenomenon to the general lessening of formality prevalent in recent years. I had observed this in my last years in college, where the younger faculty seemed to enjoy being called by their first names, giving their students a false sense of equality.

Of course the medical community dons no such mask of egalitarianism, preferring a clear-cut one-up, one-down relationship. Addressing the patient—solely because he is a patient—by a first name serves this purpose perfectly: It defines, at the outset, the role that individual is expected to play, and vice versa. It thus recreates the relationship between an adult and a child—the one dominant, intelligent, and important, the other submissive, unintelligent, and unimportant. The fact that people go along with this arrangement illustrates how willing most of us are to act like children when we are sick. I am not suggesting that as a patient (or, for that matter, in countless other situations), one should never allow oneself to be addressed by one's first name for fear of surrendering one's autonomy. Healthy or sick, an individual's autonomy should not be so fragile.

That the person at my door also *asked permission* to come in and speak with me was similarly symbolic, and no less significant. This man did not assume, like so many others, that just because I was a patient in a hospital I was fair game to *observe* and *study*, like an animal in a zoo or a prisoner in jail.

* * *

"I'm Dr. Knight. My job is to advise and guide second-year medical students. Two of them recently read about Systemic Lupus Erythematosus and have expressed an interest in learning more about this illness. I heard from one of my colleagues that you were here, suffering from a severe lupus flare. I understand you've had lupus for a long time and are very articulate and knowledgeable." He paused for a moment, as if this compliment were not sufficient, and added, "And also easy to talk to."

I looked up at him with a broad smile, as if to prove him right.

"I realize," he continued, "this is a particularly difficult time for you, Miss Szasz, being, I imagine, in some discomfort, but I was wondering if you would feel up to talking to these two students about your experiences living with lupus. I know they would be very appreciative of whatever time you could give them. And I would be happy to arrange it for a time most convenient for you, so as not to disturb your rest."

I was completely taken aback by this request, and considered saying, "I'm sorry. You know what I've been through recently. I really don't feel like talking about it any more." I had reported my "history" countless times to countless people since my admission to the hospital. Dr. Knight would have apologized for disturbing me and that would have been the end of it. I was tempted to decline. But I didn't. Maybe I did have something to offer these students beyond the cut-and-dry clinical accounts of lupus they had read. I also felt I would be talking to them because of what I *knew*, not simply because of what I *was*, a hapless lupus patient. After all, there probably was no shortage of lupus patients for them to "examine." Or they could have read, without my knowledge, my own hospital chart, which was, after only eleven days, nearly as large as a textbook on lupus. And if they had just wanted to *see* the specimen described in the text, they could have tagged along on the doctors' hospital rounds any morning.

"I wouldn't mind at all, Dr. Knight," I said. "You know I have lupus, but you may not know that I'm a librarian. Of course, I'm tired of the 'history' telling expected around here, but I've missed being able to help students with real questions."

I tried to balance my private pessimism (which I like to think of as realism), with my public light-heartedness and sense of humor. I agreed to meet with Dr. Knight's students the following evening, after dinner and after the 6:30 evening news on television. I could have skipped what the hospital called food, but didn't want to miss Peter Jennings.

* * *

The medical students arrived on time and were as polite as their advisor had been the evening before. One was a young woman, the other a young man.

"Hello, Miss Szasz." It was the young man who spoke first. "How are you feeling tonight? Dr. Knight told us this might be a good time for you to see us. As you know, we're second-year med students. I'm Dr. Warren and this is one of my classmates, Dr. McDonald."

Only second-year medical *students* and already they have been trained not only to *think* of themselves as doctors, but to *call* themselves doctors. Evidently not very comfortable with the pretense, Dr. Warren added, "Please call me John."

"And I'm Karen."

"And you may call me Susan," I heard myself saying, not without some second thoughts. I had to be several years older than these student-doctors, but being addressed by them as "Miss Szasz" made me feel old, in that odd way I feel when old-fashionedly polite students address me as "ma'am" in the library. Besides, I think of Susan as my professional name, almost as formal as Miss Szasz.

There was only one chair in my otherwise modestly comfortable private hospital room. Neither of these well-mannered students were so presumptuous as to sit on my bed, but instead scrounged the halls for another chair. "Try to find two if you can," I called out as John headed towards the door. I decided I'd feel more comfortable, too, if I sat in a chair. If the three of us were going to talk about *living* with lupus, I saw no reason to remain lying in bed.

Returning to the room dragging two chairs, John again opened the conversation. I sensed that Karen was shy. I wondered if her reserved manner had something to do with her greater susceptibility to, and hence fear of, the disease that stared her in the face. While Dr. Knight had warned me of his students' minimal knowledge of lupus, I was sure they knew that between eighty and ninety percent of all cases occur in women, typically striking in their late twenties.

"We've read about lupus, but haven't seen anyone who has the disease. I'm sure you know that currently there's a lot of interest in autoimmune diseases, and we've been taught quite a bit about the scientific aspects involved. But we'd like to hear from you how having an illness like this has affected your life. I don't really know where you want to begin. Can you remember when it all started?"

I took a deep breath. "I guess you know enough about lupus to understand that what I am going through right now is a 'flare.' But I've been living with lupus for more than fourteen years. It all began in the summer of 1968. I'd just turned thirteen. . . ."

I looked at John and Karen. If they were second-year medical students, I figured they were probably twenty-three or twenty-four. As I sat there recalling the events of that summer, I thought perhaps they were doing the same. We were all a bunch of kids having a good time at the beach.

Two

When I was younger, I could remember anything, whether it had happened or not.
—Mark Twain

Something told me this would be the last August I would spend on Cape Cod with my mother, father, and older sister. As it turned out, I would be right, but for only half the right reasons. I suspected that by this time the next year my parents would be separated. No more family vacations. No more "family," as I had known it. That change in my life, however disruptive, I was fully expecting. Actually, by this time, I looked forward to the dissolution of our small family unit. My parents were not getting along. No vacation could get us away from that. While I do not believe in the increasingly popular theory that stress causes illness, it is, of course, not impossible that circumstances prior to 1968 played a part in the onset of my illness. As I see it, other events played a more important role in what was to come.

Parental tension aside, for me it was a pleasant enough time. A cottage on Cape Cod was a part of our summer routine I had always enjoyed. We stayed at the same spot on the beach every year, close enough to the tip of Provincetown to walk to town, if you really wanted to, much of the way along the hot white sand. My sister, Eva, and my father shared this interest. My mother and I did not. This was only one of the many patterns created over the years, each of us relaxing in our own distinctive ways. My father always brought his typewriter along, and spent a good part of the day at "work." Although he enjoyed the outdoors and the hot weather, the idea of just sitting out in the sun was completely alien to him. My mother spent a good deal of time indoors as well, cooking fabulous meals as she always did, enhanced by the fresh seafood we rarely ate at home. She was less driven than my father, so it was not aversion to inactivity that kept her from lounging idly on the beach. It was her skin. She had vitiligo, a type of "hypopigmentation," the absence of the color-producing pigment, melanin, resulting in pale spots on the skin. Its cause is not known. While not directly related to lupus, there would later be speculation that my mother's vitiligo might have had some connection with my developing lupus. Whenever she went outdoors she always sat under a large beach umbrella, dressed in loose-fitting, long-sleeved garments and a hat. For as long as I could remember, she'd always had blotchy skin—milky patches over her face, arms, and legs, quite noticeable even on her otherwise fair-toned complexion. She was extremely adept at disguising these blemishes with makeup, from head to toe. Watching her perform this elaborate routine regularly, I learned the value of looking well— for oneself as much as for the outside world. The more she was exposed to the sun, the more numerous the spots became, and the more they turned from pale to sunburned in color.

If anyone in the family was determined to get her money's worth out of these beach vacations it was my sister. Then fifteen (going on twenty-one), Eva spent most of her time sprawled out on the sand, or, when more ambitious, digging huge, elaborate trenches, all the while attracting the attention of every male between the ages of thirteen and thirty plus. And how she tanned—just as effortlessly! It wasn't fair. She looked more than good enough with her normal coloring. Now there was one more thing about her for me to envy.

My sister and father both tanned quickly and deeply. My mother just sunburned. I never seemed to do either. This year, I was determined to change that and get some color. I rationalized that the only reason I went home each year as palefaced as when I arrived was because I didn't spend enough time trying to get a tan. Actually, I never liked the idea of simply lying around soaking up the sun. I didn't mind short walks out to the sandbars to catch starfish, or going for a swim in the buoyant salty water, but if I stayed out too long I always got a headache. I would soon return indoors to a book or the television.

This year, I tried to break the pattern. Vanity won out over good sense. I decided that all I had to do was persevere. I got up one morning, put on my bathing suit, grabbed a towel, and followed Eva outside. I spread out my beach towel so I could lie down on my stomach. Maybe

I'd fall asleep in this position, making the time go by more quickly. I looked at my watch. No moving for at least two hours. The morning passed faster than I expected. Before heading inside for a bite to eat, I dove into the water for a short swim. After lunch, but before returning to my towel, I looked at myself in the bathroom mirror to assess the progress. There was none. I guessed I'd have to persevere a little longer. I went back outside. The afternoon went by considerably more slowly. It was hotter, the sun was stronger, and the headache I had always "listened" to was telling me it was time to call it quits. Instead, I turned over on my back, so I would tan evenly. This position didn't do much more for the tan than any other; it only increased the pain in my head. I felt as though I were frying my brains out. Still, I was determined to see at least one day through on this new regime. If I could get through day one, the rest of the week would get easier.

When I saw Eva late that afternoon walking towards the cottage I knew it was time to follow. Browner still than the day before, she was beginning to look like one of Gauguin's models. All we needed were palm trees. As I ran up to meet her she gave me more than her typical disdainful glance, but restrained herself from telling me how awful I looked. I figured she was just ignoring her kid sister. Once inside, I went back to the mirror. I sure didn't look like my sister (one couldn't hope for a miracle in just one day), but I did have some color. I was BURNED. As red as the Cape Cod lobsters we were about to eat.

By the evening, I could tell this was no ordinary sunburn. My skin didn't hurt as much as everyone around me expected it would by the way it looked. Nevertheless, I diligently spread some chic apres sun cream all over my body. I think I was still more interested in following my sister's example than my own common sense. Several hours later, shortly before going to bed, I started to feel a little strange. I got up again for one last look in the bathroom mirror. My feeling "puffy" was not my imagination. My face, especially around my eyes, was swollen. My nose felt stuffed up. I came out into the living room and confessed to my father that I didn't feel so great. At thirteen, I was intimidated, even scared, by my father. Still, he always listened to me, and Eva, more than my mother. And he understood. He also worried more. Now he had an especially troubled look on his face as he went to get me an antihistamine. After listening to a short lecture on overdoing it, I took the Pyribenzamine he handed me and promptly conked out for the night. I went to sleep pleased, nevertheless, that at least I had succeeded in changing my skin color from white to red, determined to try for a better shade the next day.

I was stunned, and dismayed, when in the morning, still groggy from the antihistamine but somewhat decongested, I noticed that my arms, legs, and face had returned to their normal, nearly white, color. All that time spent in the sun had been for naught. I felt stupid for having wasted a day on a senseless exercise in vanity. If I couldn't look as pretty as my sister, maybe I could pride myself instead on having better sense. Never again, I thought. Little did I know then that I would never again spend another day of my life lying on a sandy beach.

I quickly put this incident out of my mind and spent the remaining days of the vacation indoors where I had always preferred to be. I was more interested in following the news of the Russian invasion of Czechoslovakia or helping my mother prepare a new recipe or finishing the Faulkner novels on my assigned summer reading list. Soon we would pack up and return home to Mansfield, a long day's drive. I was eager to return to school the next month. I was a good student and loved school, and luckily the feeling was mutual. I may have wished I was more athletic and more attractive, but I learned early to cultivate my natural talents and try to reconcile myself to what I lacked. More than ever, I now had good reason to immerse myself in my schoolwork: What better way to shut out the tension between my parents than by studying behind my closed bedroom door?

* * *

The first month of the new school year went by uneventfully. I was in eighth grade at the same private school I had attended for the last six years. The classes were small, the teachers were competent, and I had made some good friends. I felt I belonged at Forest Academy. As for life at home, it had gotten no worse.

One cool morning in October I awoke and noticed that my hands felt stiff. It hurt to open and close them. But after one of my typically long, hot showers, the pain seemed to go away. I didn't give it much thought. Several mornings later the pain in my hands reappeared, this time accompanied by stiffness and pain in my knees as well. I racked my brain for an explanation, and managed to find one. Forest Academy had a demanding athletic program consisting of an hour-and-a-half of physical education every day: field hockey and gymnastics in the fall, softball and archery in the spring. I had probably been clobbered in the shins by a hockey stick or had pulled a muscle in a futile attempt to mount the balance beam gracefully. In addition to these plausible causes for my aches and pains, my sister and I had resumed our usual figure skating activities, after time off for the summer. I was just out of shape, had overdone it, and had strained something. It sounded good to me. I didn't feel *that* bad. I kept it all to myself. Except for spending longer and longer in the shower each morning, no one at home could have noticed anything unusual about my behavior.

Slowly, my discomfort intensified. The more in shape I got, the worse the pain, especially in my knees. This was no longer a matter of overdoing it. And even if I could continue to explain away the pain in my knees, why were my hands so stiff each morning? Something was definitely wrong.

* * *

My memories of medical experiences before this time were quite limited and, for the most part, like those of any other teenager. I'd had the measles and the mumps, but not the chicken pox. My sister and I, like most siblings only a few years apart, tended to pass bugs back and forth. We also shared in the habit of not hiding our ailments from our parents when we didn't feel well. However, when it came to ordinary sore throats (which were often detected even when we chose to hide them), the response in our house was hardly commonplace. I can remember, with less than the fondest of childhood memories, that whenever Eva or I so much as *looked* as if we had a sore throat, my father would mysteriously appear out of nowhere with a culture stick in his hand, ready to take a sample to the laboratory at Mansfield General Hospital, where he worked as a professor of psychiatry. He had taught Eva and me to open our mouths so wide he could see all the way down to our esophagi without using a tongue depressor. The downside was that he also insisted that his repeatedly stabbing the culture stick deep into our throats was the only way to get a good sample.

I had been in a hospital once, when I was about four, for the croop, and vividly remember the cold air of the oxygen tent, but nothing more. I can recall visits to the ear doctor, usually for swimmer's ear. My routine visits to the dentist were mildly unpleasant, but my teeth were good and nothing special was ever done to them. I never envied Eva's braces! And then there was the eye doctor, Dr. Drysdale. My experiences with Dr. Drysdale, very early in my life, taught me more than I realized at the time.

I couldn't have been more than three when I first went to see the ophthalmologist. I still remember the big leather chairs and beautiful oriental carpets in his office. I liked going there. It was an adventure to go downtown, to a building that seemed as large as the Empire State. I always went with my mother and remember feeling like a VIP as we pulled into the valet-parking garage and rode the attended elevator to Dr. Drysdale's office on the fifteenth floor. I felt I was expected to act older than my age—I had to learn the alphabet carefully so I could read the eye charts on the wall.

Unfortunately, my eyes didn't work very well. Not only did I need glasses because I was farsighted, I also had what is commonly known as "lazy eye," or, more technically, amblyopia. I didn't particularly mind the eyeglasses. I was too young even for kindergarten, where other kids might make fun of me. Besides, everyone said I looked cute with glasses. I was also too young to realize that cute doesn't mean pretty. But the eye patch for my lazy left eye was another matter. I tried several models and found one worse than the next. The standard patch, nothing more than a large round bandaid, made me look like a pirate and took half of my eyebrow with it every time I removed it. Soon I was introduced to a new and improved version that clipped to the inside of my eyeglasses. Somewhat more comfortable, but with less than a tight seal, this model made it easier to "cheat." I began to wonder why I was going through this.

After only a few visits to Dr. Drysdale, a routine began to emerge. I always came with my mother, but I saw the doctor alone. My mother stayed in the waiting room. This was okay. It was easy to like Dr. Drysdale. He was about the same age as my father, but much less forbidding. He always had a big smile on his face as he greeted me with his usual, "Suzabelle, how are you today?" lifting me up onto the high chair that I still need a hand to reach. He spoke in a soft, deep voice, never saying too little or too much for me to understand. He seemed to take an immediate liking to me. I came to think of him as an affable "old man," a sort of Santa Claus, but thinner.

Dr. Drysdale made me feel comfortable. And I reciprocated with affection and candor. I confessed to two "sins": I had memorized the order of the letters on each row of the eye chart and could recite any given line regardless of my ability to read it. As long as I could estimate the size of the letters, I knew the correct sequence for the entire row! And I was either not wearing the eye patch at all, as I was told to do for all my waking hours, or I had been "cheating," peering out from the edges of the patch, pacifying those who wanted to see me wear it while at the same time allowing me to see. While Dr. Drysdale repeatedly encouraged me to wear the patch, as did my parents, no one tried to force me.

I never regretted not cooperating with this treatment. Patch or no patch, I would need to wear glasses. The patch would correct only one problem, which was mostly cosmetic. If I was going to end up wearing glasses anyway, why subject myself to the discomfort? The scientific reason, that the images of the two eyes might "fuse," I learned later, was unlikely. No doubt that's why neither Dr. Drysdale nor my parents pushed me to comply. While I wasn't in school yet, it wasn't all that far off in the future. There I was certain to encounter more than my fair share of teasing for the glasses alone, without the patch. Dr. Drysdale could easily have tricked me into believing the patch would cure me. But I would have soon discovered I'd been misled, only to distrust him in the future.

I had no way of knowing how important these first medical experiences with Dr. Drysdale would become later on in my life. Needing eyeglasses, even at the age of three, was not that big a deal. But, like any other first impression, these were important in setting the stage for how I would view subsequent medical encounters. There probably isn't a child in America who doesn't remember his first trip to a doctor or a dentist. Unfortunately, most do so because of the associated unpleasantness, if not outright fear. I was spared this, and not merely because my father is a physician. From Dr. Drysdale I learned a very important lesson: While a doctor might be able to help—in this case by prescribing glasses—he cannot always fix what is wrong.

Sadly, I think, children are taught to think of doctors as special people with special expertise, special authority, and, most important, special powers. They are taught to do what doctors tell them, just as they are taught to do what their parents tell them—unquestioningly. Many people never outgrow this sort of blind obedience to authority. Like children, they simply prefer to be taken care of.

* * *

After several weeks of increasingly intense pain in my hands and knees, I knew it was time to give in and see a doctor—one other than my father. While I had not completely hidden my complaints from my father, he had gone along with my wish to ignore them—for a while.

It all began effortlessly with a house call from a pediatrician who also happened to be a neighbor and a colleague of my father at Mansfield General. I had met him before, not as a patient, while walking in the neighborhood. My sister and I never really had a "kid doctor" for routine checkups. My father had always kept a medical eye on us, even giving us the standard vaccinations and filling out the health questionnaires required for school. We were both normal, healthy children; there never seemed to be any reason to go to a doctor.

Until now. But now it was not at all clear to whom I should go. So my father asked Dr. Patterson to come see me. A tall, thin, reserved man, Dr. Patterson's manner might have seemed aloof to most kids my age. But I tended to find inaccessible adults more intriguing than intimidating. Dr. Patterson appeared rather distressed on that first of many house calls. Not by my condition, which showed no outward signs and was hardly alarming, but by the larger-than-life-size poster on my bedroom door of Richard Nixon emblazoned with the words "NOW, MORE THAN EVER!" Actually, there wasn't too much Dr. Patterson could do. He had a limited private practice, spending most of his time as a hospital-based physician and in research; at thirteen, I was slightly past a respectable age for a pediatrician; and perhaps most important, Dr. Patterson had no idea what was wrong with me.

* * *

Monday, October 28, 1968. The first of many referrals to specialists, this one to the chairman of the Department of Preventive Medicine. I had no idea why I should be seeing someone in "preventive medicine."

But there were several good reasons why I went to see Dr. Hauser: He and my father were not only colleagues, but also good friends; both had done some of their training at the same well-known midwestern medical school; and Dr. Hauser, despite his departmental affiliation, was a nationally recognized expert on infectious diseases and an amateur expert on rheumatic diseases.

With the exception of an occasional visit to my father's office, I had never been inside Mansfield General before. My father's office didn't look like it belonged in a hospital anyway. There was no evidence of anything medical in the Department of Psychiatry, just a lot of lounge chairs, sofas, and ashtrays. Lots of ashtrays, always full of half-smoked butts. Now I was seeing an entirely different wing of the hospital. My father and I entered the elevator in the lobby. It stopped one floor up, and an orderly wheeled in a patient on a stretcher, intravenous bag hanging at the side. This wasn't like going to the eye doctor at all. Instead of beautiful oriental rugs, I was now seeing the ugly side of illness and medical practice. The real stuff. I wasn't scared, but I knew this was serious. My father introduced me to Dr. Hauser and left for his office.

Dr. Hauser was older than my father (my only gauge of adult age at the time) and had an air of importance about him. Behind his staid manner and solemn look, however, I knew there lay an attentive eye and a heart of gold. His grey hair and slightly overweight build softened an otherwise stern posture. Not quite old enough to be grandfatherly, he nonetheless displayed that winning combination of looking tough on the outside while being soft on the inside. He was easy to talk to—mainly because he listened.

I described my symptoms as clearly as I could, focusing primarily on the peculiar stiffness in my hands and knees. It was my first experience explaining pain to a physician. Describing any symptom in a clear and credible manner can be difficult, pain especially so, because it is so intangible and invisible. Only as it relates to doing something, or not being able to do something, does pain take on any meaning understandable by someone *other* than the person in pain. I told Dr. Hauser how I awoke each morning, noticing first that my hands were stiff and wouldn't bend at the wrist. Sometimes the pain caused simply by opening and closing my hands woke me up in the middle of the night. My knees were similarly stiff, especially in the morning. Other than taking longer, hotter, showers—which helped some—I had not been doing anything for the pain. No medication. No restriction of activities.

"Once I get going in the morning, it doesn't bother me much later on in the day. I've never felt like this before. And it seems to be getting worse. It certainly isn't going away."

Dr. Hauser spent a long time "manipulating" my joints—hips, knees, shoulders, elbows, neck, fingers. He moved joints I didn't even know I had. He said very little as he worked his way through my anatomy, as if the silence would help him hear something. But he didn't know what was wrong with me, and didn't pretend to. That didn't mean he offered no advice.

"I want you to take three aspirin, four times a day. Twelve aspirin, every day," he began.

That seemed like a lot.

"Aspirin can be hard on the stomach, so be sure you eat something with each dose."

I liked to eat—I was a good twenty pounds overweight—so telling me to eat didn't require any encouragement.

"I'm sure you've never taken this much aspirin before," he continued, "and it may be too much. Fortunately, your body has a way of telling you when you've taken too much—you'll experience a ringing sensation in your ears. I don't want you to be afraid of taking too much. If you can tolerate twelve a day, I think it will help. But I want you to tell me if your ears start ringing. Okay?"

I took the aspirin as directed. About a week later my ears began to ring. Actually, it felt more like buzzing than ringing. I was determined to be precise.

* * *

Physicians like to talk about the need for their patients' "compliance," and they like to complain about their patients' "noncompliance." Most doctors, however, are unwilling to admit how often they fail to discuss adequately the course of treatment with which they expect their patients to comply. As a rule, they do not explain what they are doing during a physical examination, what they are looking for when they order certain tests, or what side effects may result from the drugs they prescribe. Presumably they conduct business in this guarded manner for fear their patients will focus on the side effects of the treatment, thereby increasing the likelihood of noncompliance; or worse, for fear of putting ideas into their patients' heads that otherwise might never have occurred to them, thereby encouraging reports of nonexistent symptoms. Apparently they assume that the less patients know the more likely they are to comply with medical advice.

To be sure, some people prefer not to be told everything. They only want to be told what to do. They want to go to the expert to have the problem fixed. Both doctor and patient thus encourage and accept a paternalistic relationship. While I don't like blind dependence on authority, medical or any other, this may—for acute illnesses or injuries—be an acceptable basis for a doctor-patient relationship. But for the treatment of chronic illnesses a relationship based on such dependence is doomed from the word "go."

The sensible alternative to childish acquiescence is, of course, not mindless antagonism to medical authority. After all, the physician is working for you, the patient. You hire him, and you can fire him. You can trust him, or distrust him. The sooner you learn to trust those physicians worthy of trust, the better and more intelligently you will be able to work with them. If a person suffers from a chronic illness—*any* chronic illness—he must learn to take care of himself and use the physician as a trusted advisor; and the physician must accept and trust the patient as the individual with primary responsibility for the management of his own illness. In order to carry out his job to the best of his abilities, the doctor certainly has a right to expect compliance, that is, cooperation. But he has an equal responsibility to provide the necessary information and support to ensure such compliance. Similarly, the patient has a right to be informed about his disease and the procedures and drugs used to manage or treat it, but also has a responsibility to comply with the *agreed-upon treatment*. Both parties to this contract must accept their responsibilities, and not focus solely on their rights, or this complex relationship, like a marriage, can deteriorate and end in divorce.

* * *

My appointment with Dr. Hauser was finished. Next on the agenda was my first experience as an outpatient in the hospital's clinical laboratory. The regular visitors' elevator didn't even stop on the third floor where the Department of Clinical Pathology was located, seemingly hidden away from the outside world. I wasn't the only visitor on the staff elevator, but this would be my first glimpse at the inner workings of a university hospital, and the first of many illustrations of how the system caters to the staff, not the patients.

When the doors opened on the third floor, everyone seemed to be heading for the same destination. The others looked like "regulars," so I decided to follow behind. As each of us approached the receptionist at the desk, I heard the same questions repeated over and over again: "Which physician ordered this laboratory work? What kind of insurance do you have?" There was a robot-like tone to the dialogue, the questions asked of the regular customers as well as of the newcomers like me. Actually, determining who was going to pay usually came first. I was covered under my father's Blue Cross/Blue Shield plan, a commonplace arrangement among most private health insurance companies, providing coverage for the employee's dependents (at least until the age of eighteen, and beyond that, as long as the dependent is a full-time student).

I took a number and waited for the laboratory technician to call it. The only other establishment I'd ever been in that used this system was the bakery in town. There, I was always eager and in a hurry, like everyone else. Here, there was no similar sense of urgency. Everyone acted as if time didn't matter, as if they had no place better to go. I learned two things during these (soon to be frequent) waits in the *waiting* room: Assume you'll be there a long time and bring something to do to pass the time; and take the time to examine the lab "slips" from the doctor, making note of the names of the tests ordered (along with any others that seem intriguing). Doing something while waiting distracts you from feeling ill. Understanding your own lab work involves you in managing your illness more intelligently. Dr. Hauser had told me, in a general sort of way, what tests he was ordering; here were the specifics, in black and white, the names of all those tests he had rattled off but which I could never have spelled. Now I could look them up, and follow up my appointment with Dr. Hauser with my own homework.

Scanning the Outpatient Laboratory Requisition, I found the names of dozens of tests, grouped together under four major categories: Chemistry, Hematology, Microbiology, and Urinalysis. Dr. Hauser had checked off something under each. Could I copy them all down onto another sheet of paper before my number was up, without being caught in the act? Not that I was doing anything wrong. I felt, however, that it was best to do my research discreetly. Under Chemistry, the boxes for albumin, blood urea nitrogen (BUN), creatinine clearance, and total protein were all checked off. Under Urinalysis, a check mark for "routine." That sounded straightforward, even if I had no idea what they were looking for. Under Hematology, checks for complete blood count (CBC), platelet count, and sedimentation rate (ESR), the "e" for erythrocyte. Lots of abbreviations. I wondered if these were standard, and if I would be able to find them listed this way in one of my father's medical textbooks at home. Under Microbiology, only one check, for rheumatoid factor. I also noticed another acronym: LE cell. It wasn't checked off. I had enough homework for one day. I had no way of knowing that this would be the test that would soon become all-important. I didn't even know it stood for "lupus erythematosus cell," discovered by three physicians at the Mayo Clinic in 1948. The test is less widely used today, having been superseded by more sensitive measures of lupus activity.

"Twenty-seven? Who is twenty-seven?"

I had become so engrossed in my work I'd nearly forgotten where I was. As the lab technician took the requisition slips from me, she gave me a puzzled look, seeing I was alone. I was on my own until I was finished for the morning; then I'd meet my father in his office and he'd drive me to school. No big deal. I was used to people thinking I was much younger than I was. In my teens, I did whatever I could to lessen this reaction. By not dressing like a child, by not having my parents with me unnecessarily, I figured I had a better chance of being treated like an adult. At least like the young adult I was.

The technician scanned through the list of check marks, gathered together empty vials for the blood, and wrote my name and outpatient number on each. There must have been a dozen by the time she finished. The stack neatly arranged, she finally said something.

"First time here?"

Maybe I did look a little nervous. I'd been doing perfectly well —until I saw all those vials. It wasn't fear of the needle, or of being stuck in a vein. I just couldn't believe anyone had that much blood to spare!

"Yes, it is. How come you need so many tubes?"

"Each test only needs a little blood. But it's going to several departments in the laboratory. Besides, we don't want to make you come back too soon."

She was trying to make me feel better, but it still seemed like a lot of blood to me. And I had a feeling this first visit was not going to be my last anyway. She took a long rubberband-like strap and tied it tight around my upper left arm, between my elbow and my shoulder.

"Make a fist," she instructed. I could see the vein bulging. Before I knew it, she had stuck the needle in and the blood was gushing into the first of the tubes. There was barely enough time for her to add, "This will sting a little bit."

From that very first stick of the needle, I have always watched every move during medical procedures performed on me, never turning my head away for a second. I suppose I react to them the way some people do to horror movies: They watch intently, even though they are revolted or frightened by what they see. I do just that with my illness, and everything that surrounds it.

Bloodwork done, the lab technician reached for a small plastic cup. "We need a urine sample. The bathrooms are just outside the door, to your left. Bring it back to me when you're done. And then you can go home."

I wished I could have gone home. But the patient role was over for the day. It was time to get to school. Despite the foreboding air around me, I didn't feel sick. I didn't want to be sick. I wasn't going to act sick.

* * *

In the meantime, I went to school as if everything was normal. No one there knew otherwise. I wanted to keep it that way as long as possible. A week later I returned to Dr. Hauser and learned the results of that first series of lab tests. Nearly all of those first tests came back— as I soon learned the technical phrase—"within normal limits." Along with the routine urinalysis, the tests checked off under Chemistry also examined my urine to detect possible kidney malfunctions. Albumin (one of a group of simple proteins found in blood serum) usually indicates kidney disease if present in the urine. An increase in the blood urea nitrogen (BUN) level suggests decreased renal function. And large amounts of creatinine (one of the nonprotein constituents in the blood) are found in advanced stages of kidney disease with the creatinine clearance test. My blood work was equally unremarkable, but at least I now knew what each test was for: hemoglobin (an iron protein substance manufactured and stored by red blood cells, which pick up oxygen as blood passes through the lungs, delivering it to tissue cells throughout the body); hematocrit (the percentage of blood cells, mostly red, comprising the total blood volume); and white cell count (a measure of five different types of white blood cells, which help fight infections and are often elevated when there is an infection or inflammation in the body). I also had a sufficient number of platelets (particles essential for the clotting of blood).

"Most of your numbers look pretty good . . . but your sed rate is quite high." Dr. Hauser spoke to me as if he assumed I was familiar with the term.

The sedimentation rate or ESR (erythrocyte sedimentation rate) measures how rapidly red blood cells (erythrocytes) fall to and settle at the bottom of a specially marked tube within a specified period of time. An abnormally high sedimentation rate does not identify any specific disease, but is frequently elevated in rheumatoid arthritis and other autoimmune or connective tissue disorders.

"Since you also showed a positive titer in the rheumatoid factor," he continued, "you might have the early symptoms of rheumatoid arthritis. But the titer was low. We really can't be sure of anything just yet. We need to wait and see."

I was relieved that *most* of my tests were normal. However, being told that my joint pains *might* be due to something as *real* as arthritis mitigated any lingering feelings I might have had that I was imagining, or exaggerating, my symptoms. My relief quickly turned into puzzlement. Wasn't arthritis something old people got? Surely there was a better way to appear grown up than to have a grownup's illness!

I told Dr. Hauser about the buzzing in my ears, carefully noting, perhaps only as children can, the distinction from the ringing he had predicted. "Should I continue to take the aspirin?" I asked. "As much as I can stand?"

"Well, aspirin should help control the inflammation in your joints that's making them feel stiff," he responded. "Until we know more specifically what's going on, I think you should keep taking it. As long as it isn't really bothering you."

So much for what I should do. What shouldn't I do? Regardless of how achy I felt, as long as it didn't interfere with my daily routine, I had no reason to *act* sick. Still, I realized I wasn't well. I didn't want to do anything that might aggravate the situation. Although I was afraid to hear Dr. Hauser's answer, I asked my last question for the day.

"I'm not sure if I told you, but I've started ice skating again this fall, three or four times a week, a couple of hours each time. Is it all right if I keep doing that?" Why someone with joint pains would want to spend time in a cold arena is another question. I wasn't even that good at it. I suppose I wanted to keep up with my skating as a matter of principle: I didn't want to *give up* anything I didn't have to.

With hardly a pause, Dr. Hauser smiled at me and said, "You can do whatever, and as much, as *you* feel up to doing. You know better than I do how you *feel*."

When I look back, permission to continue ice skating should not have been as important to me as it was. But there was something about Dr. Hauser's response that struck me then, and has remained with me to this day. Without any clear idea about what was wrong with me, he did not impose the sick role on me and pretend to "treat" me by *forbidding* things.

As a result, I decided not only to do *as much* as I felt capable of doing, but to do *no less*. The only way to discover how much I could do was to push myself, to the limit. Doesn't everyone go through life doing just that? I assumed, perhaps naively, that most people did. I was wrong. But I learned something else, back then: If you are healthy and push yourself to succeed in life, you are called an overachiever, sometimes scornfully, often enviously. But if you are sick—especially chronically sick—and push yourself to succeed in life, like a normal person, you are called courageous, sometimes pityingly, more often admiringly. It may be one of the few benefits of being chronically ill: You score points where others don't, sometimes just for being alive.

* * *

In November, Dr. Hauser told me I could do whatever I felt up to doing. Unfortunately, my father was much more protective and much less permissive. He refused to allow me to accompany my friends to a Nixon rally, a week before the election. My heart had been set on this. But the weather had turned cold and rainy. My father's assurance that his vote would count more than my presence at this event didn't make me any happier.

I knew I was getting sicker, but I kept up my normal schedule, trying to prove, mainly to myself, that I was okay. I couldn't deny the pain in my joints, even if I tried. I just didn't want to act as if I were really ill, yet. It was a brave attitude for a thirteen-year-old girl, I suppose. But it couldn't last. I found myself, with increasing frequency, either in a doctor's office or in the hospital outpatient laboratory, repeating descriptions of my aches and pains and giving what seemed like gallons of blood and urine.

My symptoms and lab findings remained unchanged for the next several weeks, turning into months. The only tentative diagnosis offered remained rheumatoid arthritis. My complaints, particularly of feeling sore, achy, and stiff in the early morning, certainly fit. The joints involved—knees and hands—were among the most commonly affected in "RA," and the symptoms were symmetrical—that is, equally affecting both knees, both hands. Along with my symptoms, my elevated sed rate (typically found in RA) added serological evidence to support the diagnosis. Indeed, everyone seemed determined to find more support for this diagnosis. Only one physician, my father, suspected anything else—lupus. For the time being, he kept it to himself.

There was a good deal of speculation about whether I might ever have had rheumatic fever, a disease that frequently follows on the heels of strep throat, particularly if undetected or inadequately treated. This in turn may result in inflammation of the connective tissue, often manifested by the arthritis-like symptoms I now felt. However, the very notion of my having had an unrecognized case of rheumatic fever seemed extremely unlikely, to me. I remember trying to convince the pediatric cardiologist, Dr. Nandi, who happened to be one of the few doctors who seemed most ready to dismiss *anything* I had to say, that I simply could not have had strep throat without knowing it. My dramatic tales of my father, running around the house with throat-culture sticks in hand, ready to take aim at me or my sister at the slightest sign of a sore throat, had no impact on Dr. Nandi. He displayed every stereotypical mannerism of the arrogant Middle Eastern man, showing no respect for a young woman and cocky self-confidence in his certain judgment.

"Suzy, you exaggerate. You are too young to remember such things."

I know I could have been wrong. But I knew, then, I wasn't. It mattered little what I remembered anyway. Dr. Nandi was not only convinced I'd had rheumatic fever when I was younger, in his opinion, I had it *right now*.

While I was bothered by Dr. Nandi's attitude, I took some comfort in the realization that he didn't seem to listen to his colleagues' ideas any more than he did to mine. He was adamant about his diagnosis: rheumatic fever, rheumatoid arthritis. In character, he delivered this verdict to my father at the conclusion of my appointment, having spoken very little to me at all. Dr. Nandi may have been sure of his opinion, but he convinced neither my other doctors nor my father. Both Dr. Hauser and Dr. Patterson (who had taken a special interest in me and my case, despite his limited practice) were skeptical about so definitive a diagnosis on still such meager evidence. They were not sure Dr. Nandi was wrong; they just weren't convinced he was right.

The situation became increasingly puzzling, so much so that my father finally voiced his own suspicion. Maybe, too, he was so irritated by Dr. Nandi's arrogance that, uncharacteristically, he had to act a bit arrogant himself. Although a practicing psychiatrist, he retained a keen interest in medicine and his technical knowledge was impressive. Suddenly he had a chance to make the most of his hidden talents. It was he who first suggested I might have Systemic Lupus Erythematosus. He fully accepted the possibility that he could be wrong. Of course, he knew he wasn't. More important, he wanted to participate in the medical discussion, in the management of my illness—for himself as much as to teach me by his example.

This idea was roundly rejected by all the "real" doctors. No doubt, they thought my father was just too worried; or maybe a little crazy; and definitely out of his league. They were certain he was wrong. Still, it was no trouble for Dr. Patterson and Dr. Hauser to humor my father by checking off the LE Cell box on my next laboratory slip. By now I knew what it stood for. Now we'd see if I had one. At the time, it mattered little to me what tests were being ordered. I only wanted to know what was wrong with me.

The test came back negative. But even *that* didn't stop my father from adhering to his opinion. At his continued insistence, Dr. Hauser and Dr. Patterson repeated the test regularly—like giving a child a lollipop after each appointment—every time I went to the laboratory. Each time it was negative.

November dragged on forever, which is to say that I was dragging myself around more and more. Each morning I woke up stiffer than the day before, and each evening I went to bed more exhausted. Just getting through the day was an effort. I'd never felt sick like this before. "It" was getting worse, but harder to explain. The aches and pains seemed to defy not only an explanation, but a decent description. It felt as though somebody had turned the gravity up.

Then something bizarre happened. My regular menstrual period began for the month, and it seemed as normal as ever. I had started menstruating when I was eleven, so this monthly hemorrhage was no big deal. In fact, I considered myself very sophisticated for my age, having mastered the use of tampons long before Eva. But I had always needed to use, in addition, the old-fashioned, bulky "napkins," safety-pinned to my underpants the first day or two, to stem my predictably heavy flow. This time, I seemed to need both for longer. By day seven, I was ready to buy stock in Kotex. To make matters worse, I couldn't hide the situation from the other two members of the family who might wonder why the box was empty.

Still trying to act normal, I left for the rink with Eva, barely able to conceal the extra layers of padding under my leotard-like skating dress. Our skating teacher picked us up, as usual, and drove us to the rink, nearly an hour away from Mansfield. By the time we arrived, I had to stop in the ladies' room. With considerable foresight, I had stashed a few extra napkins in my duffle bag. I discovered I'd soaked through the three I already had on. Undaunted, though slightly grossed out, I skated hard for the next two hours. Maybe I knew they were to be my last for a very long while.

We returned home late that night, the drive made slower by an early snowstorm. I barely had the energy to change for bed. Again, I had to replace the pads. I knew this was getting serious. I emerged from the bathroom and announced to my mother that I had killed the box of Kotex. My father's now permanently worried look darkened perceptibly as he overheard this bit of news. Even with this "female" problem, it was easier for me to tell him, rather than my mother, the tough part.

"I really think there's something wrong with me, Daddy. I've been bleeding for a week now and it isn't getting any lighter. Actually, I think it's getting *worse.*"

"I'd better call Dr. Klein in the morning and get you an appointment. You'd better get some rest. Don't worry about going to school in the morning."

When I awoke I was relieved to find that my mother had taken Eva to school and my father had arranged for Dr. Klein to see me—as soon as possible. In this case as in others to follow, my predicament was lessened by my father's medical connections, without which I would probably have ended up in the emergency room of the hospital or even admitted, rather than simply being the first person in the waiting room to see the doctor.

No less exhausted than the night before, I managed to get ready by the time my mother returned to pick me up. I guess it was more appropriate for her to take me to the gynecologist, but I would have preferred my father's company.

As usual, I took the effort to dress nicely for the appointment, always wanting to look my best. This time I worried lest I bleed through my clothes, ruining them and embarrassing myself. It hadn't yet occurred to me that for this appointment, unlike for most of the others I'd had so far, I would be naked most of the time.

"Mommy, can we stop at the drugstore?" I asked, breaking the silence in the car.

"We really don't have time, Suzy. Don't worry, I'll ask Dr. Klein's nurse to give you some Kotex as soon as we arrive," she responded, reassuringly. We hadn't talked much about what was happening to me, and even now she only added, "You know that Dr. Klein is my gynecologist too, don't you? He's very kind. The exam may seem awkward, but he's very gentle." My mother was trying to talk to me like a young adult, but she still made me feel like a child.

No doubt a lot has changed since 1968. Today, a thirteen-year-old girl wouldn't feel so utterly out of place in a gynecologist's office. Then, I couldn't help but feel as if everyone was staring at me, wondering whether I was pregnant or suffering from some terminal disease. Located in a building of doctors' offices, Dr. Klein's was small and stark. I guess since it wasn't *in* the hospital, I expected it to look more elegant. Like Dr. Drysdale's. There were no oriental rugs here. The waiting room was crowded, with women only. That shouldn't have surprised me, but it did. Under different circumstances, my first visit to a gynecologist might have made me think about growing up, about becoming a woman, about having sex, about babies. Such things were far from my mind. I just wanted to stop bleeding.

The nurse called me into the examining room, gave me a paper gown made for someone twice my size and the familiar plastic cup. She weighed me, took my blood pressure, and pricked my finger for a sample of blood. After all those tubes, week after week, this seemed kind of silly. But it was the routine here, and I had come to accept the idiosyncracies of each doctor I encountered.

Dr. Klein was a trim, neatly dressed man, professional yet pleasantly informal. He looked a little like Charleton Heston. He spoke continuously as he performed an examination I'd never experienced before. Contrary to stories about how terrible gynecological exams are, especially when performed by a man, the only discomfort I remember came from having to lie in an absurdly uncomfortable position: on my back, legs apart, feet in cold metal "stirrups." Before I knew it, Dr. Klein had finished his physical examination but continued to ask me how I had been feeling.

"Well, besides being tired all the time, I guess my father told you about my heavy period this month. Today's the eighth day and it feels like the first. It's a little bit scary." I had to admit it. It was.

"I don't want you to worry too much about that. It looks like more blood than it really is. I don't know what your blood tests will show, but I suspect you're anemic. That would at least partly explain your fatigue. I don't know why your menstrual cycle has gone on so long, but I'm going to give you a prescription for something to stop it. That shouldn't take more than a day or two. Let me know if it's any longer than that."

The medication, a male hormone, worked like magic. The bleeding stopped. But I didn't feel any better. I was incredibly tired, no matter how much I slept. And I was getting stiffer and stiffer. I still had enough energy to attend school, but not to ice skate. Slowly, reluctantly, I was giving in to my increasing disability.

Next to go was physical education at school. Actually, this was much more strenuous than skating, and I probably should have stopped it sooner. When I went skating I could rest when I wanted, or hang back in the penalty box and spend more time watching than working out. In PE, I had no such control. If I didn't keep up with my classmates, I risked being teased or belittled.

I recalled that Dr. Hauser had told me I could do whatever I wanted and was comfortable doing. I had. But the time had come to stop pushing myself. Dr. Patterson was beginning to wonder if I should be in school at all. The three of us negotiated a compromise: School, but no more physical education. It seemed like a fair deal.

It lasted only until Thanksgiving.

* * *

Up to this time, my monthly report cards from school showed not only a string of straight A's, but not a single day absent. November's report confirmed in writing my deteriorating health: three "incomplete" grades and fifteen days absent. Soon after my exemption from physical education, I began cutting short my school days, leaving at noon, missing Latin, algebra, and art. They weren't my favorite subjects anyway. In just two months I had gone from having a few aches and pains to being dramatically incapacitated.

Then everything quickly changed, for the worse. I had a "low grade" fever, nearly always one degree above normal. I also had generalized edema (fluid retention) and signs of cardiac enlargement. My previously near-normal lab tests began to show proteinuria (protein in the urine) and hypoalbuminemia (an abnormally low content of albumin in the blood), indicating that the disease was affecting my kidneys. On the days I didn't visit the outpatient laboratory at Mansfield General, I checked my urine at home, using the "dip sticks" my father bought at the pharmacy. Yellow was normal, with darkening shades of green indicating progressive grades of proteinuria. Mine soon became darker than anything on the package's test pattern.

I was willing to go to the hospital as often as necessary, even daily, in order to avoid *staying* there. As long as I could manage at home, I was better off running back and forth for tests. I was growing increasingly dependent, physically, on my mother. She was home more hours of the day than my father. I didn't like this arrangement, but I trusted my father's opinion that it was far preferable to "living" in the hospital. I can remember a brief period of time when my edema was so bad I could hardly squeeze my feet into my winter boots. If I had known then what I know now, I might have suggested that someone from the lab come to the house to draw blood and take a urine sample. Why that option occurred to no one else either, I'll never know. Still, difficult as they were, the trips to the hospital became my only motivation to get out of the house at all.

Despite the mounting clinical evidence, there was still no agreement on my condition. I had more pronounced symptoms and more alarming laboratory signs than two months earlier, but I had no diagnosis. Naming this mystery was not my foremost concern. For me, the diagnosis was a medical nicety. Determining the disease might satisfy the doctors but wouldn't change anything from my perspective. Whether or not I had a disease someone could name, all I knew was that I was feeling awful, couldn't go to school, and could barely walk around the house, much less go outside alone. To top it off, confined to the house all day, I had no way to escape the mounting tension between my parents. Like all children, I sometimes felt I was the cause of much of their fighting. But most of the time I knew better. Actually, their concern for me was the only common ground they shared the last year of their marriage.

While I was too sick to go to school, school came to me. I was ambivalent about this arrangement. I was bored and needed the distraction, but I hated to be *seen* by people from school. It was not that I looked so terrible. On the contrary. Except for my swollen feet and pale face, I showed almost no outward signs of ill health. As long as no one from school saw me, everyone there would assume my condition was very serious. Most of my friends' parents had already concluded I was too sick for their children to visit, no doubt assuming I must be contagious. If my teachers came to tutor me, my credibility as a sick person might be questioned. It may have been a silly reaction on my part. But it was not irrational.

The tutoring wouldn't have been so bad had it not been the most intensive in the subjects I liked the least: Latin and algebra. That was happenstance. I suppose it was good for me. The agony of translating passages from Pliny or trying to solve equations about the meeting of train A traveling at speed X and train B traveling at speed Y helped to divert my attention from the pain that was now with me constantly. I realized I was fortunate to have teachers from my own school as tutors. They provided a small, but important, link to my other life, as well as a glimpse of what I longed to return to. I kept up with most of my other classes on my own—French, English, social studies—by reading and submitting the required assignments. The only serious gap in this home education program was science. But I was more than making up for that with a crash course in medicine.

Of course, I didn't study all the time, and had plenty of time left to kill. When I had too little energy to read I began indulging in a habit I have yet to break: watching soap operas. Mindless. Passive. Stupid. But I could watch the "soaps" in my own room, on my own TV, with no one disturbing me. Insipid as these shows may seem, they provide the viewer with a sense that, no matter how bad things are, they could be worse. Not surprisingly, most of the "drama" on these programs takes place in hospitals—half the characters are doctors or nurses *curing* the other half, the patients *dying* from some dread disease. Like most other popular depictions of medicine, rarely, if ever, is the focus on someone coping with a chronic disease or disability. People are either healthy, acutely ill, or dead.

During this time of disability I was introduced to yet another form of "distraction therapy." My hands hurt more than ever. But, oddly, the more I used them, the better they felt. Never one to suggest something mindless like squeezing a tennis ball as physical or occupational therapy, my father suggested something to exercise my brain as well as my hands—typing. Always an avid and omnivorous reader, he had developed interests far beyond his own professional field, psychiatry. The philosophy of language, history, semantics, classical liberalism, and political theory—these were just some of his intellectual passions. My father's library was filled with marked-up texts by John Locke, Thomas Jefferson, John Stuart Mill, Edmund Burke, Ludwig von Mises, Friedrich von Hayek, Richard Weaver, Hannah Arendt, and too many more to mention. Not yet certain how he planned to use various passages from their works, he decided I should sort through this accumulation of quotable excerpts and type them out. The therapeutic effect of this regime on my "arthritis" was minimal. The intellectual benefit I gained from reading these works while typing from them was immeasurable. They literally opened my eyes to the world.

Just as I was losing so much of my bodily integrity necessary for independence, I was discovering how terribly important a sense of personal autonomy and individual responsibility are in one's life. Soon I was reading more and typing less. Then I could type no more. By Christmas I hit bottom: I was unable to get up and go to the bathroom by myself. No matter how objectively ill you are, or how subjectively sick you feel, *this* is what really counts. This is the point at which you, the patient, *must* rely on others for assistance with your most basic bodily functions. No matter what your age, suddenly you are an infant again. I needed mothering more than ever. And that, too, presented a problem.

As my own condition spiralled downhill, so did the relationship between my father and mother. While helping me to cope with my illness gave them a reason to stay together, it now also forced them to remain in a situation both found increasingly intolerable. Whether or not I was the cause of their problem, there was no denying that I interfered with its resolution. That this wasn't my fault either didn't matter much to me. I was beginning to want out of this "home" as much as they did. I felt caught, not only in my own predicament, but between their quickly escalating differences towards my illness.

My mother, just beginning to realize, though not accept, that Eva and I were growing up and therefore needed her less, saw my illness as an opportunity to hang on, to maintain control over at least one of her daughters, and hopefully her husband as well. As my father tried to teach me the importance of overcoming obstacles and maintaining autonomy, my mother tried her best to keep me dependent— on her. Like a hostage, I knew what I would do if I ever got out of this alive. It wasn't time to act on it yet, but I was about to make a very important decision that would affect the rest of my life. I knew my sister and I were old enough to have a say about which parent we would live with after their divorce. For me, the lines were clearly drawn: If I lived with my mother, she would "take care of me" in a way that would make me increasingly dependent on her. If I lived with my father, he would teach me to take care of myself. That was the rational part of me, weighing the intellectual merits of growing up with my mother or with my father. But there was also an emotional side: I might not have been certain of what I wanted, but I was certain of what I didn't want.

Whatever this illness was, it didn't look as if it was going to disappear completely. Ever. No one had actually said this, but by this time I concluded that if I had something that could be cured, it would have been. Since the only diagnosis seriously being considered was rheumatoid arthritis, and I knew that was chronic, I assumed I was facing something life-long. There was now also the constant worried look on my father's face, and his talking more about lupus, even to me.

Maybe I was just preparing myself for the worst. Whatever that was, I had to learn how to take care of myself.

Three

> Physicians think they do a lot for a patient when they give his disease a name.
> —Immanuel Kant

January 1969. In retrospect, I cannot understand why the possibility of my having lupus was not taken more seriously. Other than by my father, that is. The period from mid-October to mid-January—nearly three months—seemed like an eternity. A new trimester had started at school. I was still at home. The pain, the boredom, the fatigue had all intensified. There seemed no end in sight.

It was time for another trip to Mansfield General. Despite the struggle to bundle up for the snow and the thought of a long walk from the parking lot, I welcomed the prospect of some fresh air. Anything to break the monotony. Thankfully, the swelling in my feet and the extreme pain in my joints was intermittent and, if I pushed myself, I could venture outside. I left the house accompanied by my mother for an appointment at Dr. Patterson's office. I was no longer able to make my way through this maze on my own. My father walked down from his own office and met us outside the door. I assumed this would be just like all the other weekly appointments to date.

Dr. Patterson spoke first, and I sensed from the look in his eyes that he was about to say something I might not want to hear.

"I'd like to admit Suzy to the hospital . . . just for a day or two . . . to perform a kidney biopsy. That's the only way we can fully assess the extent of kidney involvement at this stage in the disease."

I sat there, thinking less about the idea of the biopsy itself—I wasn't sure what it actually entailed—than about being admitted to the hospital. That idea I didn't like at all. I had made it this far without being hospitalized a single day, one of the few comforts I could point to in this otherwise bleak situation, and one that made me believe I couldn't be *that* sick. I turned to my father, hoping to hear some scientific explanation to support my instinctively negative reaction to the suggested procedure. Hardly pausing, he responded, calmly but firmly.

"I believe a kidney biopsy would be unnecessary now. There's enough evidence from Suzy's laboratory findings, especially the massive proteinuria, to indicate significant renal involvement."

Without mincing any words about my ill health in my presence, he continued, "And there's always the risk of infection from the procedure. Given how poorly she's feeling already, I don't think it's such a good idea. Besides, you know as well as anyone that no one gets any rest in the hospital! That wouldn't be good for her either."

It sounded like a good argument to me. But it still left open the possibility of performing the procedure later, when I might be up to it. Maybe my father was just trying not to come down too hard on Dr. Patterson. While this was not the first time they had disagreed professionally about my case, they always did so politely. They liked and respected each other. Or maybe my father was saving his most telling point for last.

"What, exactly, do you expect to determine from the biopsy?" he added, as if his argument needed a summation. "Will the results in any way affect your recommended course of treatment? Unless the outcome will dictate one course of therapy rather than another, it seems to me unnecessarily invasive."

Dr. Patterson's silence indicated that he agreed. With or without the biopsy, the same questions remained: From what disease was I suffering? What treatment should I receive?

* * *

It is worth noting in this connection that while it is medically preferable to precisely identify a disease before prescribing a course of treatment for it, this may not always be possible or practical. The danger in beginning a course of treatment to alleviate symptoms is that one risks masking the disease, making the diagnosis more difficult. But withholding treatment can be frustrating for the patient, because nothing is being done. Both doctor and patient must weigh doing nothing against the (strong) possibility of doing something unnecessary—or harmful. This dilemma is particularly difficult for the patient in the early phase of a chronic illness, or later during an episode when the illness is exacerbated for some unknown reason. But if you push too early and too hard for a diagnosis, you are likely to get one. And the chances are that you will get an incorrect medical diagnosis, or, better yet, a psychiatric diagnosis. Why? Because whatever your "real" illness might be, assuming you have one at all, you are seen as overly concerned with your symptoms. Obsessed. Depressed. No one understands or believes you. If there's nothing medically wrong, you are mentally ill. You must not forget that a wrong diagnosis, like unnecessary treatment, can do more harm than good.

Growing up with a father who was a physician, I was undoubtedly more attuned to this dilemma than the average person. I was also aware of his unrelenting critique of coercive psychiatry. I knew it was in my better interest to remain patient, rather than pressing to become a "patient."

This scenario holds for many diseases that are difficult to diagnose in their early stages. It may be especially relevant to lupus. Typically affecting young women, the disease frequently begins with little more than fatigue, achiness, and general malaise. Especially nowadays, when women are expected to do more and more, complaints of this nature are often seen as malingering, regressing, copping out. If you present yourself to a doctor with these symptoms alone, and have no abnormal laboratory findings, you are likely to be told, "Oh, it's all in your head." Coworkers, friends, and family members may be as unsympathetic as physicians. Ultimately, it is up to you to decide to whom you listen: If you firmly believe you are physically ill, you owe it to yourself to take seriously what your body is telling you. If you do not think your physician is doing his job, investigating all the possibilities, you can either live with his diagnosis (or non-diagnosis) or get a second opinion, or a third. But you must remember this: In the end, getting the right diagnosis answers only the question, What is the scientific cause for your feeling ill? It won't necessarily tell you what to do about it. And if the diagnosis is one of a chronic, potentially debilitating disease, it won't be the end of your struggle, but only the beginning.

To be sure, a diagnostic label *is* important. It is not only an aid to therapy but is also necessary for properly managing many social and financial matters—for example, dealing with employers, insurance companies, or disability review boards. At thirteen, I didn't have to worry about these things. But I had already sensed the ever-present need for *credibility*—in the eyes of doctors, teachers, and schoolmates.

* * *

On January 30, 1969, I was removed from my medical limbo. Dr. Patterson and Dr. Hauser were finally convinced—by the accumulation of laboratory evidence if not by my father's persistent prodding—that I had lupus. Strangely, despite the many details I can recall up to this climax, the circumstances surrounding this pronouncement are lost in my mind. I remember the date only because of a notation in a calendar marking the first day (of what would be alternate days) on which I began taking 125 milligrams of Prednisone, a synthetic cortisone. Twenty-five small white pills every other morning. Now I understood why Dr. Patterson and Dr. Hauser hesitated for so long before making *this* diagnosis: They wanted to be absolutely certain before commencing such powerful chemotherapy—and what might well become long-term steroid therapy.

The long-awaited diagnosis *was* important. It legitimized my symptoms with an acceptable, though dreadful-sounding, label. And it helped set in motion a definite course of treatment. This was a turning point. I had survived the last few miserable months. Now I wondered what the treatment would do. Would I feel better? Would it cure me?

* * *

People expect to feel relieved when they get an accurate diagnosis for their symptoms from their doctor. This idea embodies an inversion of the adage, "No news is good news." Actually, for many undiagnosed patients, the good news ("There is nothing wrong with you") is actually bad news ("No one understands or can explain how awful I feel"). Thus, with the diagnosis comes the oxymoronic conclusion, "Bad news is good news." But despite the "good news," the patient is now expected to "grieve." This brings me to remark on the currently fashionable psychobabble about the "stages" a patient must go through to cope with a newly diagnosed disease (especially if it is chronic or terminal). According to this view, the short-lived elation from a diagnosis is immediately followed by "denial," "anger," "bargaining," and "depression." Whatever truth there may be in such a generalization, it is intellectually vacuous, and for the patient, quite worthless. Experiencing each of these emotions, in the proper sequence no less, apparently is a requirement for reaching the final stage of "acceptance." Sounds to me like the sequential rituals of religion: baptism, first communion, regular prayer, last rites. But these are not discrete emotional states one experiences only after contracting a terrible disease. Rather, they are emotions experienced more or less continuously throughout everyone's life. Assuming one passes neatly through each of these stages, what should a person do with his life once he has reached the "healthy" stage of "acceptance"?

* * *

I believe I began "adjusting" long before I was diagnosed as having lupus. Perhaps having all those months of uncertainty worked to my advantage. I knew there was something seriously wrong with me that I was going to have to live with. It developed slowly, insidiously, progressively; it didn't seem likely that it would disappear overnight, or perhaps ever. Time to think, and to learn. Having the kinds of doctors I had helped. Dr. Patterson and Dr. Hauser were not the type to keep the truth from me. And to top that, my father was also a doctor and he too believed in telling me as much as I wanted to know. They all had a mightily receptive audience. I *wanted* to know what was going on, what ailed me, what would help me. I wanted to know everything.

The term SLE, systemic lupus erythematosus, had come up months before, even when it wasn't being taken very seriously. So by the time I was officially diagnosed, I knew, admittedly still only very vaguely, that lupus was "something like arthritis." In 1969 it was also commonly referred to as a collagen disease, that is, a connective tissue disorder. The currently popular categorization as an autoimmune disease was decades away. But in addition to inflammation of the joints, the systemic nature of lupus meant that the inflammatory process could manifest itself in any connective tissue of any organ of the body. Partly for my own knowledge—but also in order to explain my illness to others— I started to read about lupus and about my treatment, Prednisone. I wanted to begin, as was characteristic in the Szasz household, at the professional end of the spectrum. I read the *Physicians Desk Reference* to currently available drugs for a description of the use and side effects of Prednisone. It was just as well I couldn't understand half of it; what I did understand sounded bad enough. I also read technical articles about lupus in medical journals I could barely comprehend. I had to rely on my father to get these from the medical school library, where he also found a 1966 textbook devoted entirely to the subject, *Lupus erythematosus: A review of the current status of discoid and systemic lupus erythematosus and their variants* by Edmund L. Dubois. I would have had an easier time if I had started with a layman's guide. Venturing outside his normal environment, my father scoured the public library. It had nothing on the subject. I had to settle for what there was. Fortunately, I had an interpreter in the house.

There were good reasons why I eagerly sought out information about my illness. Long before I ever considered becoming a librarian, I grew up believing that information was power. Having more information about lupus would not affect the course of the disease itself, but would help me manage it. It would help me to better understand what my doctors were telling me, or *not* telling me. If I wanted to work with them, I had to learn to speak and understand as much of their language as possible.

In addition to this intense intellectual motivation, I still needed to fill up all my free time while I remained home from school. The Prednisone had renewed my energy, practically overnight. I felt wound up every waking hour, and slept less and less. I read more philosophy than ever, but my father was beginning to run out of things for me to type! I needed a new subject to tackle.

As a librarian, I now have better methods of doing library research. As a child confined to the house, I had no choice but to go along with my father's style. He always began with whatever books he had in the house, and he had plenty. This primitive approach was not as bad as it may sound, but his collection could have used a little updating. One night I came across a dusty copy of *The Merck Manual*, 7th Edition (1940). My father had acquired the book during his own medical training and never threw it away. Although it no longer bears the subtitle, "A source of ready reference for the physician," it remains a standard compendium of diseases and their treatments. It seemed like a good enough place to start.

I looked in the index but discovered no separate entry for "systemic lupus erythematosus." All I could find was a general definition for "Lupus Erythematosus":

> A chronic (occasionally acute) superficial cutaneous inflammation, occurring most especially on the face, scalp and ears and characterized by slightly elevated, erythematous, yellowish or grayish scaly patches of varying sizes and shapes, tending to superficial atrophy and scar formation.

Puzzled, I read on. The third of the three varieties of "LE" described was the "primary acute type . . . associated with severe constitutional involvement (pains in bones and joints, fever, pulmonary and gastrointestinal symptoms). High mortality."

I was about to jump up and go running for my father for an explanation, but it was the middle of the night and everyone in the house was asleep. I tried not to focus on those two words, HIGH MORTALITY. Despite the ominous tone of the text in front of me, I read on, coming to the sections on "therapy" and "additional remedies." Among the recommended courses of treatment, I found: "Gold sodium thiosulfate . . . intravenously. . . . Sometimes, quinine . . . is of value; sometimes sodium salicylate or salicin." The "additional remedies" were even more amusing: "Arsenic, fulguration, high frequency current, and quartz lamp (ultraviolet light) producing acute sunburn." I wanted to laugh. Then I marvelled. How could my father possibly have recognized *my* lupus if *this* was what he had been taught? I looked at the title page of the book again. Could this really have been compiled in nineteen hundred and forty? The text was not quite thirty years old. But it was like reading something from another century.

The next day my father and I searched the house for something more, and found another dusty relic from his medical school days, the *Textbook of Medicine*, edited by Russell L. Cecil, 5th Edition, 1942. (Regularly revised and updated, this book continues to be widely used.) Encouraged by the fact that there was a separate article devoted to "Disseminated Lupus Erythematosus," I plunged in. Two things immediately caught my attention: The entry was called one of a handful of "entirely new articles on subjects not covered in previous editions," and it appeared under the category of "Infectious Diseases," specifically,

"Diseases of Doubtful or Unknown Origin." Although no more up to date, this text was a great improvement over *The Merck Manual*, providing an explanation not only of the systemic character of the disease but also a discussion of the type affecting organs other than the skin.

> Among the heterogeneous group of so-called rheumatoid diseases, disseminated lupus erythematosus constitutes a disease entity, distinguished by a prolonged clinical course. . . . In spite of its name this disease bears no relationship whatever to tuberculosis and lupus vulgaris [tuberculosis of the skin] . . . In recent years it has been recognized that the skin rash is not invariably present.

Of even greater interest for me was the description of symptoms. These, at least, seemed to match my own:

> The salient clinical manifestations are: (1) a prolonged irregular fever with a tendency to remissions of variable duration (weeks, months or even years); (2) a tendency to recurrent involvement of synovial and serous membranes (polyarthritis, pleuritis, pericarditis); (3) depression of bone marrow function (leukopenia [low white count], moderate hypochromic anemia, moderate thrombocytopenia [low platelet count]) and (4) in advanced stages, clinical evidences of vascular alterations in the skin, the kidneys, and the other viscera. . . . The pain and sometimes swelling of various joints may at first make it difficult to distinguish the condition from rheumatic fever or from rheumatoid arthritis. Suspicion may first be directed to its true nature by finding a leukopenia . . . As the disease progresses, the hemoglobin falls more rapidly than the red cell count. . . . In the more advanced stages, the blood platelet count is apt to be depressed . . . red blood cells are found in microscopic examination of the urine. . . . Small amounts of albumin are also usually to be found. The appearance of large amounts of albumin, red blood cells and casts, resembling the urinary findings of an acute glomerulonephritis, signifies the development of extensive vascular changes and of glomerular [kidney] damage. It occurs in the advanced stage of the disease and completely eliminates the diagnosis of rheumatic fever. In addition to arthralgia [joint pain] and arthritis, attacks of pleurisy [inflammation of the lining of the lungs] or of pericarditis [inflammation of the lining of the heart] may occur at any time during the disease.

Now I understood how and why my father suspected, almost from the very beginning of my illness, that I had lupus. Still, I was surprised that he remembered so much of this after so many years. Each clue in the mystery of the last three months seemed to match not only the words, but their order of appearance, on these two pages of text. Unfortunately, while the description of symptoms helped to satisfy my intellectual curiosity, the discussion of the prognosis and treatment was scarcely more encouraging than that in *The Merck Manual*.

> The fever and other manifestations of the disease may continue for many months, with long alternating periods of exacerbation and of remission. In some cases complete remissions may last for years, but the ultimate prognosis is grave. . . . Most sufferers from this disease ultimately die. . . . No form of specific therapy is available. . . . Confinement to a darkened room or one in which the windows are covered with red cellophane seems to be helpful.

I had just read in *The Merck Manual* that exposure to ultraviolet light with a quartz lamp ("producing sunburn"!) was one of the recommended remedies. To appreciate medicine one must know some medical history. Popular writings on illness and health invariably contain a warning, directed especially to readers who might be patients, *against* reading medical literature that is more than a few years old. The information, so this argument runs, is likely to be outdated and therefore misleading. Exposure to such material may unduly alarm the patient, adding to his distress. In my opinion, this sort of warning is insulting, implying that the wrong information (or even too much of the right information) is as bad for the patient as the wrong medicine (or too much of the right one), and that only the physician knows what, and how much, medical information the patient needs, just as only he knows what, and how much, medication to prescribe. But is the subject of medicine really all that recondite, reserved for experts? Thomas Jefferson didn't think so when he observed, "No knowledge can be more satisfactory to a man than that of his own frame, its parts, their functions and actions."

As for outdated information causing anxiety, would anyone seriously suggest that reading about the early misadventures of Orville and Wilbur Wright might make the reader afraid of flying? Shouldn't we all be curious about past events, beliefs, and practices—whether in aviation, religion, or medicine? Outdated medical information should be read for what it is: not misinformation, but historical information. As such, it presents—regardless of the specific disease discussed—a fascinating glimpse at scientific progress, or the lack of it. Indeed, it often reveals surprisingly little progress, especially in discovering the causes of numerous diseases, despite advances in their treatment.

The story of lupus is a good case in point. While SLE may not have the name recognition polio did in the 1950s, or AIDS has today, it is fast becoming a widely recognized and discussed disease. It is better understood and better managed than when my father went to medical school, but there is still no known cause or cure.

* * *

March 1969. Nearly two months after being officially diagnosed with systemic lupus erythematosus and commencing chemotherapy (which now consisted of Prednisone and Cytoxan, an immunosuppressive drug frequently used in patients receiving organ transplants, to inhibit rejection), nearly four months since being confined to the house on a more or less permanent basis, and over five months since the ordeal began with nothing but a few achy joints, I returned to school.

I was impatient beyond words to go back to school, to get out of the house. My restlessness (largely artificial energy from the steroids) was matched by a quick, and significant, improvement in the clinical and laboratory manifestations of my lupus. However, in addition to the positive side effect of the Prednisone (at least from this patient's point of view), one of the negatives is the general suppression of the immune system, making the body more susceptible to infections.

Even if I was physically ready, going back to school was no simple matter, emotionally. My feelings were confused and contradictory. I really didn't know what kind of reception I expected—or wanted. On the one hand, I wanted to be treated "like everyone else," "like nothing had happened." On the other hand, I craved some recognition for what I had been through, some reward for what I had successfully endured. This was an unrealistic wish.

My "healthy" appearance contributed to the problem. I went out of my way to look as good as I could. I agonized over what to wear, practiced applying blush to my cheeks to help minimize my "moonface" (puffiness caused by the Prednisone), and skillfully disguised my extensive alopecia (hair loss caused by the Cytoxan) with a hair "fall." Fortunately for me, these variations on wigs had become popular in the late sixties, and having an excuse to wear makeup at age thirteen was something of a bonus too. All in all, it was an impressive disguise but I soon paid the price for it. Looking so well was good for my self-esteem but bad for my credibility. Looking well despite being gravely ill may be a particularly insidious feature of lupus, but it is not uncommon in other chronic illnesses as well. Although I quickly grasped the problem, it would take me years to learn how to dress and make up for various occasions, from visiting with friends to seeing doctors to dealing with disability review boards.

Obviously, the few friends who had visited me at home, as well as the teachers who had tutored me, had seen me looking "sick," and were pleased to witness my "recovery." But from the vast majority of people at school, the unspoken sentiment I sensed was, "You *look* fine. You couldn't have been *that* sick to have been out of school for all this time." Maybe too, because my father is a psychiatrist, a few people probably suspected I'd really just had some sort of nervous breakdown that needed to be disguised.

Four

> Strictly speaking, the question is not how to get cured, but how to live.
> —Joseph Conrad

In June I finished the eighth grade on schedule with the rest of my class. Even better. I decided to skip a year and enter high school in the tenth grade. I had several reasons for forging ahead, besides wanting to impress people with my heroic accomplishments while ill. And were they impressed! I also had a hidden agenda. While I had never discussed, in so many words, how close I had come to dying—not with my doctors, my parents, or my sister—I knew perfectly well that it had been a strong possibility. Many critically ill people must be aware of that much. Once past such a life-threatening time, you cannot help but feel you had better get on with it because you are living on borrowed time. This sounds corny, I know, but it's the truth.

Keenly realizing how very precious time was, I didn't want to waste another minute of it. The ninth grade seemed like a complete waste of time. My skipping it after missing so much school was less heroic than it sounds. I had been tutored throughout my illness, studied on my own, and actually missed very little. Moreover, my eighth grade curriculum at Forest Academy was considerably advanced, nearly up to the level of a standard ninth grade public school program. The same was not true of the school's college preparatory program. I had known for years that my parents wanted me to transfer to MacArthur High, the public school in our neighborhood, when it came time to go to high school. Many students switched to high school elsewhere, either to one of the better public schools in Mansfield or to a boarding school away from home (if their parents were very wealthy and/or wanted to get their children out of the house). I knew I didn't belong in either category. And although I was the only one in my class to skip a grade that year, the practice was not uncommon. I just managed to score more points playing this game than my healthy peers.

In any case, I could have waited, as my sister Eva had done a year earlier, and remained in familiar surroundings. But in addition to having a sense of urgency, I also felt the need for a change of scenery. Returning to my class at the school I had attended for seven years was comfortable, providing me with the continuity and support I needed. But it also had its disadvantages, or so I felt. I thought my illness had become the primary focus of my identity at school. Until the events of recent months, I had been regarded as "Eva's little sister." While being in her shadow annoyed me, this remark was always meant in a positive sense. Eva was an outstanding and popular student. Now, instead of being in her shadow, I felt like I was in my own dark cloud, which might never blow away. I needed a fresh start, a clean slate. At a new school, I would have this. I wouldn't have to explain my past, palliate people's misplaced fears, or second guess their sympathetic gestures. As I prepared to enter MacArthur High in the fall of 1969, I concluded that the people there would know only a few things about me, not necessarily in this order: I was Eva's sister (therefore I must be smart); I was starting the tenth grade a year early (therefore I might be even smarter); I was *short*. Unlike my moonface and thinning hair, that physical characteristic I could not hide.

* * *

Getting sick at any age is no picnic. But there are advantages to facing this type of life crisis early. It may seem odd to suggest that being ill can ever be advantageous, and even odder to suggest that the earlier in life you are faced with a chronic illness, the easier it may be to adapt to it. (I am, of course, not referring to children who are too young to understand what is happening to them when suddenly struck with a serious disease.)

The most obvious but nevertheless often overlooked element that makes dealing with a chronic illness problematic is the issue of dependency. When you are sick with the flu it's nice to be pampered by your family—for a few days. And they may even enjoy showering you with special attention—for a few days. But when the illness is chronic, the pleasures of enjoying dependency—or satisfying it—sour quickly. Clearly, it is easier for children to accept the dependency inherent in the "patient role" because they are already dependent on others, especially their parents. Unlike adults stricken with illness, who have to *give up* some aspects of their independence, children have much less to *give up*. Reciprocally, the burden on the caregivers, especially parents, is less of a departure from their normal routine. To be sure, a sick child greatly increases the burden of dependency on his parents. But the change is a matter of degree, not kind. On the other hand, a young person faced with a chronic illness has to learn, the hard way, the importance of independence and responsibility, and thus comes to value them both all the more. Oliver Wendell Holmes—physician, author, and father of the Supreme Court justice—reveals the brighter side of illness when he suggests that the best way to ensure a long, productive life is to "have a chronic disease and take care of it."

But "taking care of it" includes far more than medical management. It affects how you direct your *whole* life. In this respect, too, it may be better to be faced with a chronic illness at a relatively early age, when you are more flexible and have more opportunities to adapt your life according to your strengths and weaknesses. I am not trying to make some profound sociological observation. I am only articulating what seems like common sense. Learning to live with a chronic illness, like learning a new language, is easier the sooner you are forced into it. Much can be made of the uncertainty inherent in many chronic illnesses and of how this makes it difficult to plan a life. True enough. The opposite is also true, if you make it so: Being chronically ill forces you to plan. Otherwise, you might take things as they come and let your life drift.

I would like to remark briefly here on the vocabulary we use to describe a chronically ill person's disability. In recent years, the term "handicapped" has fallen into disfavor, especially among those to whom it is attached, having been replaced by the term "disabled." Supposedly, "handicapped" has more negative connotations than "disabled." The former term does tend to conjure up the image of some visible impairment, usually physical. The term "disabled," on the other hand, implies *loss*. *Webster's* defines the condition of being disabled as the "inability to pursue an occupation because of a physical or mental impairment; lack of legal qualification to do something." As against all these negatives, the term "handicap" is defined as "the advantage given or disadvantage imposed; a disadvantage that makes achievement unusually difficult."

It is important to put one's handicap, like everything else, in perspective. If you can use your "handicap" to your advantage, you are a fool if you don't. You must not, however, use it as an excuse to avoid responsibility or demand special rights based solely on your status as a sick person. Healthy or sick, what matters in the end is not what you have lost or can't do, but what you have left and still can do.

* * *

I didn't look forward to the summer of 1969. I was ready to begin my new school year as soon as the old one ended in June. I wanted to get on with it. One important reason for my lack of enthusiasm for a vacation was the realization that I would be forced to spend more time at home. I was keenly aware of the mounting tension between my parents. Confined to the house, I had witnessed much more of it than Eva. I knew that my father had remained at home during this last year largely, perhaps solely, in order to see me through this ordeal of medical uncertainty and severe disability. He had been waiting to make any move until my condition had stabilized. It's not that he was waiting until I was well enough to abandon. On the contrary, he knew, better than anyone, that I would never be completely "well" again and would have to learn to live with my illness. And he didn't want to leave me, or Eva. He just wanted to leave his wife. I also realized that my father had to overcome his guilt feelings about leaving his wife. He could not "take" Eva and me away from our mother, so to speak, because *he* wanted us with him; it was something that *we* had to want. We had to make the choice, to assume the responsibility for deciding which parent to live with. Disrupting the routine of our family life, however strained, in the midst of my medical crisis was out of the question for my father. Besides, although I didn't know this until much later, he had stuck it out for years. A few months more didn't matter.

One hot evening that summer, my father finally announced that he was moving out. I, too, had already packed a bag and was ready to go with him. I had seen how my mother had tried to manipulate him, and I didn't like it. Worse, I had witnessed—first hand—her attempts to use my ill health to make me dependent on her, and I liked that even less. Painful as the realization was, I recognized that her inability to respect those she loved stemmed from her own lack of self-esteem. By the age of fourteen, I realized that much of her adult life had been marked by unresolved ambivalence. Born in Syria to Christian Armenian parents and educated in Beirut, she emigrated from Lebanon to attend college in America, returning only once. She felt guilt for not keeping in touch with her parents or any of her six siblings. She married in order to remain in the United States as a citizen, or so it seemed to me. She obtained a master's degree in social work from a prestigious university, yet never pursued a career. She spoke four languages—French, Arabic, Turkish, and English—fluently. Having been educated in American schools in Lebanon, her English, unlike my father's, had not a trace of an accent. And she had many remarkable talents, any of which she might have made more use of. She could tailor a dress or a suit from her own tissue-paper drawings; she could knit an intricate sweater, practically overnight, without a pattern; she could sing, and whistle, like a seasoned performer; and she could recreate any dish from any cuisine after just one taste. She could do all these things quickly, effortlessly, and perfectly. Yet it seemed as if the better she was at something, the more she resented doing it and withdrew from doing it.

I wondered whether I might have been able to help my mother change her style had I stayed with her. But I doubted it then, and I doubt it now. I confess that my own selfish interests took precedence. I took heart in some of the words of John Stuart Mill I had typed for my father: "The term duty to oneself, when it means anything more than prudence, means self-respect or self-development, and for none of these is any one accountable to his fellow creatures."

Initially, my father, Eva, and I moved in with my grandmother, who lived alone in a small house only a few blocks from us. My grandfather had died some eight years earlier. Living with her was the best temporary arrangement while my parents worked out the details of their separation and divorce. Well before the beginning of the new school year in the fall, the three of us were reestablished as a new household. While Eva and I had seen a good deal of our grandmother, and we got along well (although I felt she preferred Eva, who looks more like her than I do), living with her—in relatively cramped quarters and during a particularly stressful period—tainted the memory of that sojourn for all of us.

In addition to my parents' separation, summer brought another major change in my life: no more trips to the beach. No more sun. There is some medical disagreement, even today, over exactly how much exposure to the sun is "safe" for a person who has lupus. In my case, there was no doubt about *this*, at least. My doctors all agreed that I had to avoid sunlight *as much as possible*. In 1969, this was much more difficult, both from a social and technical standpoint, than it is today. There were no over-the-counter sunscreens on the market! Dr. Patterson had to prescribe a topical sunscreen of five per cent PABA (para-amino benzoic acid) in seventy-to-ninety-five-percent ethyl alcohol; the pharmacist had to prepare this solution especially for me. I, in turn, had to apply this lotion to all my exposed skin, repeatedly, throughout the daylight hours.

Much has changed in twenty years, medical fashions being no exception. In 1969, smoking was still popular and acceptable; there were cigarette dispensing machines even in hospitals! The same was true for tanning, the darker the better. Today the tide has turned sharply against both practices. To be sure, there are tanning salons in the United States. On the other hand, consider an item such as the feature article in *Newsweek* of June 9, 1986, entitled "The Dark Side of the Sun," and the Cable News Network reporting the next month that the dollar volume of sales for sun-screen products (*excluding* those products targeted for tanning) has risen from $37 million in 1981 to $85 million in 1985. In 1969, even pharmacists were unfamiliar with PABA as a sunscreen. Today, dozens of brands are displayed in every drugstore and supermarket.

Less obvious aspects of photosensitivity—and more difficult to explain to other people—are the many things that do not offer as much protection from the sun as one might assume: for example, clouds—which filter some of the sun's harmful rays, but do not eliminate them; water, snow, or sand—which may reflect the sun; and shade from a tree or a large umbrella—which still allows for indirect exposure. In addition, small amounts of ultraviolet light are emitted from photocopying machines, quartz lamps used in dentists' offices, fluorescent light bulbs, camera flashbulbs, and even the romantic glow of a fireplace!

Lupus patients, or anyone who wants to minimize exposure to the sun, should also wear long sleeves, slacks, and hats, and avoid the hours of the day when the sun is most intense (roughly between ten and four). My own adjunct to using a sunscreen is to carry a parasol. It offers more protection than a hat, and doesn't blow off my head—though it's boring to respond to onlookers rudely commenting that it isn't raining.

Giving up the sun didn't mean having to give up a summer vacation. Instead of our usual family trip to Cape Cod, my father took me to New York City. My first trip to Manhattan; my first vacation with just my father. It was splendid: shopping at Bergdorf Goodman; lobster salad at Sardi's, cheesecake at Lindy's; and The Theater. My father convinced me to see *In the Matter of Robert J. Oppenheimer*, and I appreciated it more than I imagined; I convinced him to see *You're a Good Man, Charlie Brown*, and he enjoyed it more than he imagined. But *Man of La Mancha* remains our mutual favorite musical, and the most memorable evening. A poignant tale of spirit and self-determination, sung most eloquently in "To Dream the Impossible Dream," struck close to home for both of us.

* * *

Fall 1969. MacArthur High. A new start, I was certain at least of that. The skeletons were all hidden in the closet. But the door couldn't stay shut very long. Whether or not I told anyone about my illness, one fact alone would blow my cover: I had to be excused from physical education. How could I explain *that*? I looked well. I was not visibly handicapped. Indeed, I had resumed ice skating, and made no secret of it. In many ways, my fifteen-minute private lessons were more strenuous than the prescribed forty-five minutes of gym class three times a week. But again there was the difference of *control*. Strictly speaking, I was able to perform most of the activities in a high school gym class, except those done outdoors on a sunny day (and who decides just how sunny it is?). When it came to skating, I could decide whether to go or not, how long to stay, and how much to rest. Obviously, this was not the case in a high school physical education class. Moreover, being unable to keep up with your peers in gym is at least as humiliating as giving the wrong answer in a math class. You can't very well say, "I'm sorry, I don't feel up to running around the track today." At least I never felt I could.

62 LIVING WITH IT

I was, in many ways, lucky to be exempt from this nonsense. I didn't have to get sweaty in the middle of the day; I didn't have to feel rotten if I was the last kid picked for a team; I didn't have to be embarrassed in the locker room for being shorter, or fatter, or fuller-chested. True, such travails are temporary and trivial compared to living with a chronic illness. But to a teenager, they can seem nearly as life-threatening.

For the management of my lupus, I continued to see Dr. Patterson, but only three or four times a year. Dr. Hauser I saw even less often. I went to the outpatient laboratory for the standard battery of blood tests and urinalyses about once a month. The lab reports went directly to Dr. Patterson, and unless they showed something abnormal, or I experienced new symptoms, there was no change in my treatment. I was definitely not in remission. I remained on high-dose steroid therapy *and* my laboratory tests continued to show signs of "disease activity." I was fortunate in that I received immense benefit from Prednisone. My symptoms, particularly joint pains and fatigue, lessened dramatically; my renal function returned to normal; and my serological signs improved too. I seemed to escape—at least for the time being—the deleterious side effects of the drug: delayed healing of wounds, increased susceptibility to infection, elevated blood pressure, edema (water retention), excessive hair growth, skin eruptions, stomach ulcers, muscle weakness, diabetes, osteoporosis (thinning of the bones), cataracts, and glaucoma.*

Strangely, I got fewer colds than before I had lupus! Perhaps this was the result of an increased awareness of my health needs, and an increased willingness to rest at the first sign of a cold or the flu instead of "fighting" it and ending up sicker, longer. One side effect of the Prednisone I noticed immediately was my increased appetite. Most of my life, I'd always loved to eat and was overweight. I lost this excess when I became ill. But as soon as I began the steroid therapy, I regained what I had lost—and then some. Maintaining a normal weight had been difficult enough for me before; now it seemed impossible. In part, this was a true side effect of my treatment. But I also used it as an excuse. Although I had many girlfriends, I was at the age when a girl is supposed to start noticing boys, and start being noticed. I wasn't.

---

*Once again, I had learned about this from reading, in this case an article by George W. Gray, "Cortisone and ACTH," in the March 1950 *Scientific American*.

But Eva was, and how. As long as I remained overweight, it was easier for me to justify, to myself, that that was the reason—rather than my being ill. Being overweight, like being ill, is a stigma. Maybe I just wanted to choose my own.

There was another side effect of the Prednisone I found annoying, though harmless: my "moonface." Chipmunk cheeks. Call it what you will. I think I was the only one who paid so much attention to it, then. And I'm probably the only one who notices it now. Generally, the side effects of the Prednisone were probably minimized because I was taking the drug on an alternate-day schedule: one dose in the morning, every other day. This is not an easy regimen to follow: I kept a calendar, so as not to mess up and take more medicine, or less, than I was supposed to.

There is good reason for taking steroids in this way. Prednisone is a synthetic derivative of the body's own natural hormone, cortisone. Under normal conditions, the adrenal glands, stimulated by the pituitary hormone ACTH, produce cortisone, which helps the body withstand stress. When you take a synthetic cortico-steroid, such as Prednisone, your body falsely assumes that *it* is manufacturing and secreting the substance, and decreases its own production. The more often you take the hormone, the more you "suppress" your own adrenal glands' activity. The idea behind alternate-day therapy, then, is to supply, on one day, the additional cortisone needed to control the disease and encourage the body to do its own job the next day. Otherwise, the body's natural process will eventually stop, resulting in a greatly increased, or even complete, dependence on synthetic replacement therapy.

Unfortunately, I was soon forced to abandon this preferred method of treatment. Although I seemed to be doing well and had no major flareups, my laboratory tests continued to show signs of "moderate" disease activity. I was also beginning to feel more achy and fatigued on the days I was not taking Prednisone. It became apparent that I needed too high a dose on a single day to get me through the next. So I began to take Prednisone daily, first once a day, then twice a day, eventually—and gradually—lowering the doses over the years.

* * *

My illness remained under control through my high school years. Academically, I was doing well, my performance not in the least affected by my having skipped a grade. However, I encountered a fresh problem that had nothing to do with my being ill: the turmoil caused by forced busing to ensure racial integration in education.

Like many other public schools in the early 1970s, MacArthur High became a center for political protests and racial disturbances. Initially, there were only minor incidents, usually confined to the cafeteria at lunchtime. Administrators tried to solve this problem the bureaucratic way: Eliminate the lunch period, cut down the time between classes, and send the students home early. Of course it didn't work. The demonstrations became more frequent and more violent. I went to school each morning at eight o'clock, ran from class to class, and came straight home at one o'clock. I figured that if I never went to the bathroom, I was less likely to be assaulted or robbed. But when my homeroom teacher was knocked unconscious and taken to the hospital at the end of my first week of my junior year, I concluded I'd had enough. How was I going to finish my last two years of high school? I had no idea. I only knew I wasn't going back on Monday.

Despite the unrest, Eva decided to remain at MacArthur High. She had only one year left to endure. And she had a boyfriend, Michael, to protect her. But several of Eva's friends had had enough and transferred to Saint Maria, one of the Catholic high schools in town. Perhaps for lack of any better alternative, that seemed like a good choice for me, too. While I played hookey for a day, my father went to speak with the nuns. They were surprised, but delighted, by his wanting to enroll his daughter in a Catholic school: No other non-Catholic parent had ever expressed such an interest before. (Today, twenty years later, nearly one-third of the student body is not Catholic.) Some of my friends were puzzled by my decision to attend a parochial school. As for my father's friends, they were appalled, and several said so. After one such "confrontation," my father—always fast on the draw—retorted, "*You* believe in integrating with Blacks. Well, *I* believe in integrating with Catholics."

After missing only two days of school, I started at Saint Maria. Until this time, my illness was the only thing that made me different from my peers. Now, I was the only non-Catholic in a Catholic school. This generated more curiosity, at least initially, than my lupus ever had.

Much like the stigma of illness, this was important for some and insignificant for others. Actually, my exemption from Mass was accepted as readily as my exemption from physical education, by my peers as well as by my teachers. Nonetheless, I suspect some parents found my presence a kind of contaminant, much as two years earlier some misguided parents thought my illness might be contagious. Soon I had more friends than ever. I liked attending Saint Maria for another reason: It was my own turf. No more being Eva's kid sister.

Soon I was approaching my senior year. Although Eva is two years older, because I had skipped a grade, she was now only one year ahead of me in school. She had stuck out her last year at MacArthur High, riots and all, and was preparing to go off to college. Partly because I was home more—not only because of my health but also because my sister had a boyfriend and a more active social life—I was conned into assuming some of the routine household chores, especially cooking. I didn't mind. I enjoyed preparing food as much as eating it. Eva allegedly did the dishes. She *also* did the chauffeuring, mainly because I wasn't old enough to drive myself. That somehow didn't count emotionally, but it did count practically. Once Eva left for college, my father would have better things to do than cart me around. I was expected to get my driver's license as soon as legally possible, which meant that my father resorted to bending the law, a little, teaching me, as he had Eva, to drive *before* we were of age—in the parking lot of MacArthur High. In the dark, so no one would see us. Driving was more a matter of practical necessity than a luxury. But, of course, for me it was, perhaps more than for most teenagers, the ultimate symbol of independence.

*   *   *

I have not mentioned my mother since I related my parents' divorce and its aftermath. It's not that I am writing her out now. In a deeper sense, I wrote her out when I decided to live with my father.

It was in the middle of July, 1971. I can't remember the exact date. The day I remember all too well. I had just returned home from a professional driving lesson. My father's patience with seeing Eva dent his own car exhausted, he bought *her* a Volkswagen bug, and *me* a real instructor. Eva was about to dash out on a date. My father was in Europe with his girlfriend—his first since his divorce, and their first vacation together. The phone rang and I answered it. I heard the voice of a distant family acquaintance. "Susan, are you and your sister going to be home for a little while? . . . I need to come over and talk to you right away." I knew something was very wrong. I knew exactly what. My mother was dead. As soon as Eva and I were alone again, we called my father and he was home the next day. Perhaps with understandable selfishness, I was relieved that this tragedy took place in the summer. Not being in school helped.

While I was shocked by the news, I was not terribly saddened. It was not that I had no feelings for my mother, no sense of having lost her; rather, it was because I felt I had already lost her. Although we lived only a few miles apart, I had seen her only once since leaving the house that hot summer evening, almost exactly two years before.

I preferred to remember her the way she was when I was a little girl: a dedicated, perhaps overly devoted, loving mother. I had already grieved her passing, her private death for me, when I went to live with my father. There was no need to do it again. Yet now, I was expected to grieve openly. I don't know how well I played the part. I did the best I could under the circumstances. We had both been through very rough times, some of it together. And just as my own struggle to cope with a serious illness made me puzzle over her lifelong lack of resiliency, so too it made me realize that only she was responsible for what she did with her life.

It made me reflect all the harder on how, sooner or later, we all experience terrible, tragic things in life. My father had. His parents had. They had fled their native Hungary for the United States, their home and fortune abandoned, barely able to speak English. They made new, successful lives for themselves. Some misfortunes we bring upon ourselves; others are completely beyond our control. But no matter what happens to us, we always have some control over what we do about it.

* * *

Looking back on my high school years, it seems as though I felt—despite my illness, my parents' divorce, and my mother's death—that I'd led a fairly "normal" life. Maybe I refused then, as I refuse now, to consider crises abnormal. Maybe I just took things abnormally in my stride. Maybe I had no other choice. I knew I could focus on these, admittedly painful, events, or on all the rest of what had happened in between, which seemed very good: the stabilization of my illness, my ability to resume ice skating, continued academic success, new responsibilities at home, and an increasingly close relationship with my father.

As the day of my high school graduation neared in June of 1972, my thoughts turned to the usual things students think of at that time: Would I go to the prom? I didn't. How well would I do on my SATs? Not as well as I would have liked. Where would I rank in my graduating class? Third—out of three hundred. Would I stay in touch with any of the good friends I'd made in only two years at Saint Maria? Only one, Kate, who is as special to me now as she was then. What college would I go to? Not the one from which I would graduate.

No one was surprised that I did well in high school. I was expected to. I wanted to. Doing well academically was very important to everyone in my family. Eva and I were both good students. Also, I realized that while my physical abilities were limited, my mental abilities were not. Although my situation was not as dramatic as that of the blind person who develops a sharper sense of hearing or touch, I used my brain to its fullest, knowing I couldn't do the same with the rest of my body. Socially, I could always fall back on my illness as an excuse to justify the time I spent at home studying, escaping the peer pressure to go out and play.

Of course, I enjoyed my success as a student. I got a standing ovation from the entire student body at the annual Senior Awards Day ceremony on June 9, 1972. There I was, up on the stage, barely five feet tall in my high heels, to accept two awards for the highest honors in English and foreign languages. When I turned around and saw everyone on their feet I almost fell off my own. Other kids in my class had received as many plaques, but not plaudits. I stood there, wondering why. The picture of myself unable to walk at all flashed through my mind. I hadn't thought about that for some time. None of my friends or teachers in that auditorium had seen me then. Only a few knew about it. I had accomplished a great deal. I had much to be proud of. I wasn't ashamed to admit it.

My father hasn't forgotten the day either. And he hasn't forgotten that I wasn't the valedictorian. Others sometimes have trouble telling when he's being critical, and when he's joking. I always know the difference.

Five

> Do not try to bend, any more than trees try to bend. Try to grow straight, and life will bend you.
> —G. K. Chesterton

At age sixteen I was, I think, remarkably immune to petty peer pressure. I'm glad I went to high school when I did. Today, graduating without ever having had a date would make a girl feel like a failure, a real freak. I always took solace in my "good Catholic" girlfriends never having had dates either.

I was not at all immune to the quite unsubtle academic family pressure with which I grew up, and which I learned to love. So when it came time for me to choose a college, it was logical that I should be seduced by an aura of academic snobbery.

I never suffered from the typical adolescent urge to leave home. Actually, many of my high school classmates remained at home after graduation, attending the local Jesuit college. It would not have been unusual for me to do the same and attend the local university. Why didn't I do that? Because Mansfield University wasn't academically prestigious enough. Stupid. Hadn't I worked hard in high school "to get the grades"? Wasn't my academic success, particularly in light of my ill health, something to be really proud of? To flaunt? I thought it was. I *deserved* to go to the best school that would accept me.

I wasn't completely stupid. I didn't apply to schools on the West Coast, three thousand miles away. I applied only to schools within a three-hundred-mile radius of Mansfield. Also, I must have had a stronger feminist streak in those days than I do now. I applied to every one of the Seven Sisters colleges (none of which had yet gone co-ed), was accepted by most, and selected one, the best. Now I possessed what

I considered to be official recognition of my intellectual capabilities—admission to a famous, first-class college.

* * *

Such eagerness for social validation of intellectual *ability* is similar to the quest for scientific validation of physical *disability*. Admission to a prestigious college proves that you are intelligent; a diagnostic label, that you are ill. If a good school rejects you, you can't be very smart; if a competent doctor can't find anything wrong with you, you can't be very sick. But the fact remains that meeting socially validated criteria is neither necessary nor sufficient for either good education or good treatment. You can be a lackadaisical student at a good school or a bad one; you can mismanage your medical treatment with or without the proper diagnosis. Conversely, you can learn as much as you want without prestigious professors and imposing architectural landmarks; and you can learn to take care of your health whether or not you are "officially" ill.

Unfortunately, I didn't have as good academic sense then as I did medical sense. I knew I couldn't get healthier simply by being treated by "experts," but I believed I could get smarter simply by being taught by "experts." I still had much to learn.

In fairness to my father, I should say here that although he contributed heavily to my being vulnerable to academic pressure, he did his utmost to disabuse me of bowing to academic snobbery. He emigrated to this country at the age of eighteen, knowing barely any English. Only two years later, having left behind his native tongue if not his cultural heritage (or his heavy accent), he applied to more than two dozen medical schools and was accepted by only *one*. And not one of great renown, the University of Cincinnati. He was rejected not because of academic qualifications, but because of a prevailing prejudice of the day: anti-Semitism. And where is he now? A professor of psychiatry at a northeastern medical school, a prolific author, and a respected public figure. I should have taken heart in his example: Do the best you can, period. While you cannot escape personal limitations or societal stigmas, you can try to succeed in spite of them. Perhaps I suffered from some kind of first-generation-American syndrome, wanting to do "better" than my parents. Perhaps I was competing with

Eva, who, very soberly, was satisfied with going to a very good, but quite unglamorous, university, not far from Mansfield. Perhaps I was just stubborn and needed to be taught a lesson the hard way.

To me, going away to college didn't seem like such a crazy idea. I seemed to be doing well enough medically. I had experienced no lupus flares since 1969 and no significant absences from school. I had as much energy as I ever did. I played a big part in helping to run the house. Living away at college couldn't be *so* different. But most of all, I was caught up in the web of my own accomplishments. I had come to cope so well with my limitations that I overlooked how precariously balanced my health really was.

What I didn't take into account, perhaps ignored, was that I continued to take a high dose of Prednisone. My feeling well was due as much to the pharmacological effects of the medicine on my psyche as on my joints. I was on a perpetual steroid "high." Nonetheless, I still showed signs of disease activity in each and every test from the laboratory. I knew I was not "well." But how was this state of affairs best described or understood? Was I in a remission? Certainly not. Was the disease suppressed? Somewhat. Was it under control? More or less.

* * *

In September of 1972 I left for college, a four-and-a-half-hour drive from Mansfield. It was three times as far away from home as my sister had gone and a lot more time in the car for my father to curse the trip, never mind worry.

Soon after I arrived, I had a brief appointment with one of the physicians at the health center. Although he had a detailed letter from Dr. Patterson in front of him, he asked me for a "history," concluding with an inquiry concerning the types and amounts of medication I was taking. He seemed satisfied with my report. Actually, he seemed stunned that I was sitting there, and expressed some apprehension about my ability to tolerate my daily chemotherapy: 60 milligrams of Prednisone and 125 milligrams of Imuran, a highly toxic immunosuppressive drug used primarily in organ transplant patients. Why was I still taking these drugs?

In lupus, the normal immune response—the body's natural defense mechanism against foreign substances, typically microorganisms causing disease—goes awry. The normal functioning of the immune mechanism depends on the body's having the necessary antibodies, acting in the appropriate fashion. For as yet no known reason, lupus causes the body to produce an excess of antibodies—*antibodies that mistakenly attack the body's own tissue.* Hence the current classification of lupus as an "autoimmune disease." The only way presently known to control the disease is to counteract this misguided attack. However, the drugs that reduce the autoimmune response also interfere with the body's resistance to infections. Imuran and Prednisone suppress the immune system, and thus control the lupus. When taken in combination, the effect is frequently enhanced, and the patient may be able to take less steroids and thus be protected from some of its harmful side effects.

No wonder my father strongly opposed this mad adventure: 60 milligrams of Prednisone and 125 milligrams of Imuran every day! My chemically controlled state was hardly suited for someone living with fifty other young women, some of whom were sniffling with a cold or the flu at all times. I must have been out of my mind. Not that I should have been treated like the "boy in the bubble," sealed away in an artificially controlled environment. I couldn't very well spend the rest of my life avoiding other people. Being at college away from home didn't seem any more dangerous than being in school and living at home. I saw what I wanted to see. I was blind, and very stubborn.

Woodland Hills College was more than just a good school, although it certainly was that. I still remember my sense of awe when I realized the entire student body of approximately twenty-five hundred women came from the very top rank of their high school classes. It was also a tremendously socially oriented school, and very traditional. Everyone was expected to attend candlelight supper on Thursday evenings, tea and bridge on Friday afternoons. At the same time, there were no required academic classes at all, the only exception being two semesters of physical education. A bit unfortunate for me. This time I chose not to be excused from sports. Why? Because I hadn't quite outgrown wanting to be like everyone else; and perhaps also because I could choose the sport to fulfill my requirement, and one of the choices was figure skating. There was still one small hitch: I had to take one semester of swimming or pass a swimming test before I could participate in any other PE course.

I hadn't been in a pool in a couple of years, but I had been an excellent swimmer. It was one of the few things I was better at than Eva. I still remember learning to swim at the age of five, attending a special class at the YWCA, the water level in the Olympic-size pool lowered for short kids. Taking a swimming class several times a week for nearly four months seemed like a waste of time. I was sure I could pass the test. How difficult could it be to swim a quarter of a mile and tread water for ten minutes? I watched as the other girls started—and some couldn't finish. I said to myself, "You know, you don't *have* to do this. You could easily *get out* of this." But I didn't. Somehow I found the strength and the stamina to pass. Strength and stamina, yes. But still not much sense.

Actually, this test had no ill effect on me. On the contrary, it gave me a sense of accomplishment, a feeling of equality with my healthier peers. It took several more days before I realized that, such irrelevant triumphs aside, this whole arrangement was beyond my powers of physical endurance. My effort was doomed to failure. Living, eating, studying, and trying to sleep in a noisy house full of strangers, instead of the pace of my own routine and the peace and quiet of home; the strain of long walks from class to class; the inescapable social pressures that became physically stressful as well—all added up to a burden I knew I could not bear, and had no reason to bear. I was beginning to recognize that stress can be both intangible and cumulative. It would be easy enough to conclude that I was simply homesick, like nearly everyone else; that I could have stuck it out; that I should have stuck it out. Perhaps. I'll never know.

Maybe I took advantage of my ill health and used it as an excuse to return home only a few weeks after I'd left. I arrived at my decision to return home quickly and firmly. I saw no reason to drag my feet once the situation became clear to me. The sooner I confessed to my mistake the better. First of all, I feared that if I was really getting as run down as I felt, prolonging my stay might result in a serious relapse. And I knew that the sooner I returned home, the more likely I was to be able to enroll at the university there—Mansfield University—without losing a whole semester. Bad enough to lose face. No point in losing time as well.

I went away to school because my pride got the better of my good sense. Coming home was an admission of failure. Moreover, it was a wholly self-inflicted failure, the result of my own decisions and actions. Some people—I hesitate to call them friends—reacted to my return with a sense of disappointment combined with disapproval. My father welcomed me back with a warm and loving "I told you so." He knew that my going away to Woodland Hills College was the wrong decision, but felt he ought to let me make it. He was relieved to have me home in one piece. I now had to come to terms with what seemed like a huge setback, psychologically more than physically. I don't regret having tried, however foolish my effort may have been. Sometimes you have to learn from your own mistakes. To this day, whenever I make a new one, my father cannot resist reminding me of this episode —as if I could ever forget it.

The comforts and constancy of life at home were, however, marred by a fresh problem: I had to find a new doctor. Dr. Patterson, whom, by this time, I would have outgrown anyway, had left town for a position at another university. I was sorry to see him leave. I had grown extremely fond of him, and he of me. He was a fine man: aristocratic in bearing, reserved in manner, utterly devoted and loyal to me, and to my father as well. We had come a long way together. I was losing a close and trusted friend as much as a doctor.

Several things come to my mind in this connection: the pros and cons of teaching hospitals; changing doctors by choice or out of necessity; the advantages and disadvantages of having an expert-specialist as a regular physician.

Many good things can be said about teaching hospitals, and I am not about to ignore them. They are likely to have more sophisticated laboratory facilities; to be more up to date concerning advances in diagnoses and treatments; and to have more highly trained physicians. But there are plenty of negatives as well. Because of the internal pressures of the profession, these highly trained physicians often stay at one institution only as a stepping stone to the next, more prestigious position. This is not their fault. It is the way the system works. Without such personal drive and institutional pressure for advancement, there would be less professional excellence. One goes with the other. The net result for the patient is not at all clear.

Although the arrangement serves to benefit the patient in search of a diagnosis for an elusive ailment, it may not be as helpful for the patient needing long-term care for a chronic condition. Like it or not, the management of a known chronic illness is not very interesting and promises little glory for the physician bent on making his mark in the profession. Finding a good doctor is never easy. In some cases, it may be preferable, or necessary, to see a specialist; in others, the specialist's expertise is unnecessary and unproductive. Specialists tend to be more interested in the disease than in the patient.

Here I was, then, back at home, back at the familiar outpatient laboratory at Mansfield General. But, by circumstances beyond my control, I was thrust into a new doctor-patient relationship. Without a doubt, Dr. Patterson would have understood my returning home from college as well as my father had, for he too had a context of successes within which to place this failure. Instead, my leaving Woodland Hills College became the focal point for Dr. Patterson's successor.

Right from the start, Dr. Rozen and I just didn't hit it off. He was about the same age as every other doctor I'd seen to date, but acted older, grumpier, and uninterested. On my first appointment, he sat staring at my thick file, barely acknowledging my presence. Aside from the lab report in front of him, his initial impression of me was based entirely on my inability to make it away from home. Indeed, it was only the "numbers" that proved to him I was really "sick." It was not an auspicious beginning. Actually, Dr. Rozen never said anything about my returning home, but he didn't have to. He just made me *feel* like a wimp.

I shouldn't have taken Dr. Rozen's attitude so personally. He struck me as someone who didn't care much about anything in life, least of all his medical practice or his patients. Despite his indifference, he managed to project an air of professional arrogance. He was overweight, but objected to my being so. He had no sense of humor. He was distant. The "discord" between us, if that's the right term, was very low key. I had not yet grown so irreverent as to deny him the respect I accorded all my elders.

Luckily, my medical condition remained stable. I didn't have to see much of Dr. Rozen. Anyway, there was no need to rely on his medical judgment in a crisis: There was none. And while I didn't "see" Dr. Hauser anymore (due to his own diminishing practice and health), his presence loomed in the background. He kept in touch with my father, and an eye on everything and everyone at Mansfield General. Last but not least, my father was watching over me, and everyone who took care of me. Maybe all this, too, bothered Dr. Rozen. He wasn't really "in charge."

People rightly believe a positive attitude about yourself is important for maintaining good health. For me, a negative attitude about Dr. Rozen helped even more: I stayed remarkably well while under Dr. Rozen's "care"!

All, however, was not bleak. Since it was barely the end of September, I could still enroll at Mansfield University, a few miles from home. I had missed only a month of classes. So what if that constituted one-fourth of the semester? I was smarter than the average student there, wasn't I? That was my main reason for not wanting to go to M.U. in the first place. No one at the university questioned my ability to make up the lost time. The people at the admissions office knew I had just returned, unexpectedly, from a nationally recognized women's college. My having left there on a "medical leave of absence" aroused more sympathy and understanding about my health than suspicion or uncertainty about my academic potential. I wish the people at the parking office had been as understanding.

Mansfield University is a huge school, spread out over a vast campus, with the typical parking problems. Virtually no one is allowed to drive onto the central campus, much less park there. But the university was required by law to provide handicapped parking permits for those eligible. But try to explain a handicap no one can see, and one you, yourself, try to hide most of the time. Of course I had the necessary statement from Dr. Rozen, indicating that I required a parking place as near to my classes as possible, to minimize both the exertion from excessive walking and my exposure to sunlight. I should have sent my application through the mail. Appearing in person didn't help. The skeptical look I received from the director of the parking office was then compounded daily by the quizzical stares I received from passersby as I emerged from my bug, parked within a few feet of the chancellor's Mercedes. Their faces seemed to ask, "Who is this VIP. She doesn't even look old enough to *drive*?"

* * *

By the spring of 1973 the disruption of the fall was behind me and I was ready for my first full semester at college. I was happy to be back home. I liked it at home a lot, something most teenagers apologize for. What was there not to like? I shared a comfortably-sized house, close to the university and also to my grandmother's house, with my father. He was often away, leaving me entirely on my own. I had my own car, Eva having turned over the keys when she left home for college. I had enough money. I had my own checking account, which I rarely used. I preferred foraging my father's bookshelf for Jefferson Davis's *Letters*, where he always hid a stash of tens and twenties.

My sister, now a sophomore, came home often on weekends, whereupon I would, with jocular hostility, announce that the house was not big enough for three people. Actually, it was a large three-bedroom ranch house with a den. Eva still had her old room, even though she also had a near-palatial apartment in Lansing, thanks to my father's generosity. I should have learned from my sister's experience as a freshman at college: Why go away to school and share a tiny cubicle with a stranger who probably smokes or snores, or both, in a large, noisy dormitory? Why engage in forced, time-consuming, often mindless social activities? Why eat unappetizing institutional food in a cafeteria? Why should *I*—living in a home that was not merely tolerable or pleasant, but positively great—do all this? Now, my sister envied *me*. For once, the tables were turned. I had a legitimate excuse to reject the peer pressure and social expectations to go away to college. I might have been "suffering" from a chronic illness, but she was suffering the hardship of life away at college, relieved only by regular respites at home. Now that I was back home I felt as though, of the two of us, *I* had the better life. I am sure Eva often thought so too, especially at the end of her weekends at home. It wasn't just my gourmet cooking that prompted her to say, as we waited for her to catch the last Greyhound back to school, "You eat like this *every* night?!"

Aside from the fact that she didn't need to stay at home as much as I did, she had a better reason, academically, for going away to a "better" school. She planned to go to medical school, and Mansfield University was not particularly strong in the sciences. For me, on the other hand, it was absolutely ridiculous to go away. I wanted a prelaw and political science concentration, subjects for which Mansfield University was nationally known. It was, however, better known for its basketball team. Still, I knew there were plenty of good teachers, too. I set out to find them.

I was never strong in math or science. I loved reading and writing—and yet, or because of that—I had an intense dislike of most required

LIVING WITH IT   77

English courses. They seemed to take the fun out of literature, dissecting novels as if they were formaldehyde-preserved frogs, teaching you how to write "academic-ese" instead of plain English. Seeing no way out of freshman English other than taking an honors class—filled with fewer students, but more hot air—I chose instead to take a series of minicourses. I would need more of them, but with each one shorter, I figured they'd be more tolerable. Despite my expectation to dislike them, I stumbled on one which genuinely appealed to me—"Southern Women Writers." Sandwiched between Carson McCullers and Eudora Welty, whose names I recognized even if I had not yet read their works, I came upon an unfamiliar author, Flannery O'Connor. I was captivated by the strange characters in her stories, but it was the life of their creator that irresistibly caught my attention and has held it fast ever since: Flannery O'Connor had lupus. She died from the disease when she was thirty-nine years old. But how had she lived?*

* * *

Born "Mary Flannery" on March 23, 1925, in Savannah, Georgia, O'Connor grew up in the South, the only child of Regina and Edward—distinguished and well-established, but not wealthy, Catholics. Initially employed as a real estate dealer in Savannah, Edward O'Connor eventually established his own business, the Dixie Realty Company. Forced by the Depression to give it up, he secured a position for himself with the Federal Housing Administration as a zone real estate appraiser. In 1938 he moved his family to Atlanta. Two years later, due to ill health, O'Connor moved his family again, this time to the home of Mrs. O'Connor's family in Milledgeville. Then, in 1941—at the young age of 44—Edward O'Connor died from disseminated lupus, the same disease that later killed his daughter.

Flannery was fifteen when her father died. She completed high school the following year and, remaining close to her mother, enrolled at what

---

*A fine account of Flannery O'Connor's life and work can be found in the "Chronology" of her *Collected Works*, edited by Sally Fitzgerald (Library of America, 1988). *The Habit of Being*, a collection of O'Connor's letters published posthumously and edited with an introduction by Fitzgerald (Farrar, Straus, & Giroux, 1979) is the source for subsequent references.

was then the Georgia State College for Women, located a block from her home. Despite her early interest in becoming a cartoonist, she earned her degree in social science. She then applied for and received a fellowship to the highly regarded Writer's Workshop at the University of Iowa, providing her with free tuition and a sixty-five-dollar stipend per term. In 1946, her first short story, "The Geranium," was accepted for publication in *Accent*, and she obtained a fellowship from the English Department at Iowa. In two years she earned her master's degree, came in touch with people with literary connections who helped her gain access to publishers and grants, and became a guest at the prestigious Yaddo Artists Colony in Saratoga Springs, New York.

Leaving Yaddo in 1949 for New York City to work on her writing, Flannery met the poet and translator Robert Fitzgerald and his wife Sally, with whom Flannery began to share much of her work and her time. After living with the Fitzgeralds for about a year at their Ridgefield, Connecticut, home—where she was working on her first novel, *Wise Blood*—Flannery became seriously ill. A local doctor thought she had rheumatoid arthritis. In 1950, on her way home for Christmas, her symptoms grew alarmingly worse. At Emory Hospital in Atlanta, she learned, in the spring of 1951, that she had lupus. She continued to work on her novel while in the hospital. After being discharged, she moved to "Andalusia," the farm outside Milledgeville her mother had inherited. During 1951, as successive drafts of her novel went back and forth to friends and critics, Flannery went in and out of the hospital. By year's end, she had spent weeks completely bedridden. Nonetheless, she completed *Wise Blood*, wrote and sold several short stories, and began work on a new novel. As if this were not enough for someone so sick, Flannery applied for and received a two-thousand-dollar fellowship from the *Kenyon Review*. The money went to pay for books, blood transfusions, and ACTH (adreno-cortico-tropichormone). As her literary output increased and her lupus began to stabilize, Flannery felt she could travel, if only to visit friends. But by 1953, her condition deteriorated and she was forced to use a cane. Still, she took her illness in stride.

> I have a disease called lupus and I take a medicine called ACTH and I manage well enough to live with both. Lupus is one of those things in the rheumatic department; it comes and goes; when it comes I retire

and when it goes, I venture forth. My father had it some twelve or fifteen years ago but at that time there was nothing for it but the undertaker; now it can be controlled with the ACTH. I have enough energy to write with and as that is all I have any business doing anyhow, I can with one eye squinted take it all as a blessing.

During the last ten years of her life, Flannery received a second Kenyon Fellowship, two O'Henry Awards (for two of her short stories), grants from the National Institute of Arts and Letters and the Ford Foundation, and two honorary degrees (from St. Mary's College and Smith). She also published a second novel (*The Violent Bear it Away*, in 1960) and nearly three dozen short stories—an unbelievable output, even for a healthy writer. Occasionally she ventured outside Milledgeville to attend readings or travel the lecture circuit, although her letters (published posthumously in 1979) suggest these jaunts produced more physical fatigue than intellectual stimulation. While recognition came fairly early in her literary life, monetary rewards did not follow suit. In 1954, she received a mere $1.35 in royalties for *Wise Blood*; a year later, a $1,250 advance for her second novel; and in 1961, $750 for her short story, "Living with a Peacock."

While Flannery's illness increased in severity, her genius blossomed. In 1955, after four years of ACTH injections, she began to take Meticorten, one of the early oral cortico-steroids. That same year the degeneration of her hip joints worsened (a frequent symptom of lupus and a common consequence of steroid therapy), forcing her—she hoped temporarily—to use crutches. This remained a permanent handicap. In 1958, Flannery and her mother embarked on an extended tour of Europe, including a trip to Lourdes—as a "pilgrim," she insisted, not as a "patient." By 1959, the necrosis affecting her bones had spread to her jaws, requiring large doses of aspirin. She could barely eat. Eventually her jaw and hip problems were attributed to the steroids and Flannery tried to reduce the dosage. Of course, it was too late to do much good for her bones. Instead, the change had a detrimental effect on her lupus. She investigated potential surgical procedures for her hips, but all had to be rejected as too dangerous in her condition. She settled for periodic injections of cortisone directly into the hips, which gave her temporary relief:

80   LIVING WITH IT

> What they found out at the hospital is that my bone disintegration is being caused by the steroid drugs which I have been taking for ten years to keep the lupus under control. So they are going to try to withdraw the steroids and see if I can get along without them. If I can't, as Dr. Merrill says, it is better to be alive with joint trouble than dead without it. Amen.

Although she bought an electric typewriter to save her from having to pound a mechanical one, Flannery claimed that she could not create on it! In the summer of 1963 her lupus flared again, this time in the form of severe anemia. In February of 1964 a fibroid tumor of the uterus was diagnosed. Despite the risk, surgery was scheduled and her cortisone dosage increased as a precaution. The operation was a "success," but Flannery developed a kidney infection from which she never recovered. On May 21, she signed her last literary contract, for a collection of stories entitled *Everything That Rises Must Converge*. The next day Flannery returned to the hospital, where "she hid[es] unfinished stories under [her] pillow lest she be forbidden to work on them." On August 2, 1964, Flannery slipped into coma and she died the next day.

I shall not discuss Flannery O'Connor's literary works. Instead, I want merely to note the astounding quantity and quality of her literary output, virtually all of it produced *after* she became seriously ill. Moreover, Flannery had to bear the added burden of suffering from lupus when little was known about it and little could be done for it. Her disease apparently never went into remission; rather, she learned to live with its unrelenting, if occasionally quiescent, progression.

Flannery's early years in Iowa, Saratoga Springs, and New York City suggest that, had she not become ill, she might not have returned to or lived out her life in Georgia. Perhaps it was her good fortune, then, to be "forced" to return home to the South, whose rich culture was a source of her inspirations.

> This is a Return I have faced and when I faced it I was roped and tied and resigned the way it is necessary to be resigned to death, and largely because I thought it would be the end of any creation, any writing, any WORK from me. [But] . . . it was only the beginning.

To be sure, had Flannery not been able to retire to Andalusia, and had she not had her mother's constant support, she might not have been able to cope so well, or so fruitfully, with her illness. Her deep faith in the Roman Catholic religion was also a great source of support for her. Indeed, her Catholicism, like her illness, was an important part of who Flannery O'Connor was.

As I write and think about this now, grateful for one of my own quiescent phases of lupus, I only hope that, in my own way, I can live up to one of Flannery O'Connor's critics' beautiful observations about her: "Of course, she lived with this illness all the time. She lived with it in such a way that she enabled people to forget about it entirely."

* * *

Curiously, if not for the fateful accidents of history, another young woman might have become an even more famous lupus patient—namely, Nikita Khrushchev's younger daughter. As it happens, the only available account of her life and illness appears to be a short essay by A. McGhee Harvey, "Medical Mission to Moscow."*

In September 1969, Dr. Harvey, a well-known professor of medicine at The Johns Hopkins University Medical School, was summoned by telephone to Moscow. His mission: to see a thirty-two-year-old woman with systemic lupus erythematosus. The patient was said to have kidney involvement, "needed" a renal biopsy, and was expected to have no more than six months to live. A friend of the family, whose identity was as yet unknown to Dr. Harvey, decided to seek medical advice in the United States. The doctor learned the identity of "his" patient only two days before his departure in October 1969. Revealingly, he never refers to her by name: only as "the patient" or the "younger daughter of Khrushchev."

Despite the urgency of the call, Dr. Harvey spent his first two days in the Soviet Union as a tourist, sightseeing. Only on the third day did he—and Mrs. Harvey, who had accompanied him—meet the whole Khrushchev family, *except* the daughter-patient, who was in the hospital. They discussed politics, toured the grounds of the Kremlin, and took extensive photographs. No one even mentioned lupus until day

---

*The Pharos, Fall 1982. This is another discovery I owe to my father and the absurd amount of time he spends reading. All subsequent references to this story are from this account.

four, when Rada, Khrushchev's older daughter, escorted Dr. Harvey to the Kremlin Hospital. To Dr. Harvey's dismay, he soon discovered that while

> all of the indicated laboratory procedures had been performed . . . there was no way . . . to judge the quality of the results other than to note that the values in some instances differed significantly from those found in [his] own laboratory.

Dr. Harvey examined the patient, whose English was good enough to give her own medical history, and found nothing unusual. She was taking Prednisone (Dr. Harvey doesn't say how much) and said she felt reasonably well. After his initial visit—which was also his last and only visit with the patient—Dr. Harvey was taken to another hospital, to see the patient's nephrologist. So far, Dr. Harvey had not discerned—either from his own physical examination of the patient, or from the laboratory findings made available to him—anything to confirm the diagnosis of renal involvement or the prognosis of imminent death.

Two more days of tourism followed. At the end of the first week, a conference at the Kremlin Hospital was scheduled for Dr. Harvey with the nephrologist and the patient's doctor, plus an interpreter. After some discussion, "all reached an amicable agreement about the current status of the patient and what should be done in the future." Where, in heaven's name, was the patient while all this was going on? Dr. Harvey also met Mrs. Khrushchev, who "asked very penetrating questions and [made] it . . . clear that *she had no confidence* that the Russian physicians would pay attention to [Dr. Harvey's] recommendations about future management of the case." Two years later, in September 1971, Dr. Harvey noticed a picture of the patient in an obituary of her father. He thought that "she looked to be in good health." Less than six months later, however, "a reporter browsing through the cemetery in Moscow came upon a small tombstone with the patient's name on it."

Khrushchev's daughter must have had access, far beyond that of any ordinary Soviet citizen, to the best medical care the Soviet Union had to offer. Yet it is clear, from what little can be gleaned from this story, that her best interests were never of much concern to her doctors. Dr. Harvey, the great expert from the West, spent more time with other physicians than with the patient.

Intrigued by this story, I wrote to Dr. Harvey, hoping he would be able, and willing, to provide me with some additional details. He declined my request, giving as his reason his desire to protect the doctor-patient relationship. But by his own accounts, Dr. Harvey saw the patient only once, and that briefly. He never even calls "his patient" by her own name. Yet, now, long after she has died, he is reluctant to say anything more about her, allegedly to protect her. From what?

Whenever I hear criticism of Western medicine—typically contrasted with glorifications of nationalized health care in socialist countries—I have only to reflect on these two case histories to draw my own conclusion.

* * *

During this time, my lupus was not in remission, but was well controlled by the steady regimen of Prednisone and Imuran. I was gradually taking less Prednisone, although I cannot remember exactly when each change of dose was made, or how much I was on from year to year. Living at home obviously agreed with me. I was medically stable. Aside from a sprained ankle—from tripping in a snow-filled pot hole, not ice skating—I was doing better than ever. I began to take it for granted that I would always be living with it this well. Perhaps too much so.

Like toward the end of high school, as I neared the end of college I began again to believe that I could do anything I wanted. Fortunately, my ability to mess up by over-reaching was matched only by my ability to promptly dig myself out of my self-created holes, try again, and succeed on my next, more sober, move. "Life," said Robert Louis Stevenson, "is not a matter of holding good cards, but of playing a poor hand well." These words seemed to have become my guiding motto.

Early in my junior year at M.U., I discovered that the university offered a special "three-three" program in conjunction with its law school. You could begin your first year of law school after three years of college, and receive a bachelor's degree a year later. This was for me. I had been planning for years to major in political science and philosophy and go to law school. I was genuinely interested in these subjects, and still am. My ambition was also strongly influenced by family pressure. Medicine and law were considered the only professions worth pursuing. This was never actually stated in the Szasz house. It was simply a given.

There was also my fondness for skipping (what I considered) superfluous grades. Nor was I about to surrender in the competitive struggle with Eva, who had just started medical school on a similarly accelerated program. My plan would allow me to graduate from law school the same year my sister would graduate from medical school! Last but not least, I could stay at home while continuing my studies. I had made *that* mistake once. I wasn't about to make it again. I thought I had learned a lot. I had. But still not enough.

So there I was, barely twenty, in law school. Much as I had wanted this—and I wanted to go to law school more than *anything* (the more so the more people told me I'd hate it)—I quickly realized it just wasn't right for me. My main dissatisfaction with law school was that the training process required to become an attorney turned out to be quite different from "studying the law." I was interested in the latter, but it was clear that I would receive little of it in the classroom. Secondly, "making it through" law school seemed to require more physical stamina than intellectual prowess. True, unlike medical students, law students are not subjected to "rounds" at absurd hours or required to make "life and death" decisions. But they, too, are subjected to an endurance test—albeit one that lasts only three years. The realization that I was engaged in a stress test, with a "law practice" as the final destination, suddenly struck me as physically overwhelming and intellectually uninspiring. Could I blame "the system" for my blindness to these blatant truths? Of course not. I can only blame myself. Once again, my desire to prove something—mostly to myself—blinded me.

The stress of law school—like any other stressful event, especially if it extends over months and years—deserves some further comments. My law school experience illustrates something I had been told over and over again but did not yet understand well enough. Along with exposure to ultraviolet light and infections, I knew—from my readings as well as from repeated reminders from my doctors and my father—that "stress" can precipitate a lupus flare and hence ought to be kept to a minimum. But readings and reminders are abstractions. Moreover, to me, as I think to most people, stress means a *bad*—unpleasant or unhappy—situation. Since I wanted to go to law school, looked forward to it, and enjoyed what I considered to be its major component, studying, how could it be stressful? The important thing about stress, however, is not whether "it" is painful or pleasurable, but the demand it places on the human body and the person as a whole. For me, the stress of law school seemed, rightly or wrongly, too great. Also, the pot at the end of the rainbow looked to be filled with something more like tarnished copper than the gold I'd envisioned.

Fortunately, it was much easier to "leave" Mansfield University Law School than to leave Woodland Hills College. Logistically, it couldn't have been simpler, in fact. I only had to re-register in a different division of a large university, walk to a different building for classes each day, and complete my senior year, like any normal college student. Still, once again, I had to "explain" to some people an admittedly sudden, and perhaps seemingly rash, modification to what I had claimed was a well-thought-out decision. Existentially, this shift was painfully difficult, far more so than switching college campuses. I had to re-think and re-plan the rest of my adult life. What was I going to do when I finished college? For years, the answer had been so obvious that I hardly gave it any thought. With my family background and upbringing, the range of acceptable choices seemed quite limited. Inevitably, I would do something academic, whatever that might mean. Teaching —college, not high school, of course—was now the next most logical option. For me, that meant philosophy or political science.

With law school behind me, I began to think about graduate school. That's not quite true. I expected it would happen on its own. In some sense, it did. I took for granted I would stay at Mansfield University, and knew I would be accepted to its graduate school. Indeed, because of my dual major and my outstanding academic record, I was pursued by not one but two departments on campus. Without asking, I was offered *two* attractive fellowships. As if these incentives weren't enough, I was also awarded a prestigious fellowship from the Intercollegiate Studies Institute, named in honor of the twentieth-century conservative philosopher Richard Weaver. As I passively accepted the notion of being a (now well paid) student for four more years, I should have listened more attentively to one of Weaver's insightful aphorisms: "Ideas have consequences."

In May of 1976 I graduated as salutatorian in a class of over five thousand. Not bad, with or without lupus.

Six

When you arrive at a fork in the road, take it.
—Yogi Berra

By late spring 1976, the disappointment of the previous semester had become a dim memory. Indeed, I managed to celebrate my graduation for several weeks after commencement. I had no plans to work during the summer. I wanted a break before resuming another four-year stint of studying. Even I hadn't yet figured out a way to get a PhD any faster.

I spent my first month off from school planning my sister's wedding at the end of June. Eva and Michael had been dating steadily since high school, so their decision to marry came as no surprise. Neither did my helping with the arrangements. I had "helped" Eva and Michael from the beginning. The first time she invited him to dinner, she hid me in the kitchen to do the cooking. Now I was addressing three hundred invitations, selecting the menu, booking a band, and ordering flowers. My father also helped, but I was responsible for most of the details of the arrangements. He paid the bills, of course. Eva didn't even pick out the cake. The best bakery in Mansfield was in the worst part of town. I insisted that Michael come along on that mission. The owner was distressed by the bride's absence, convinced that she would be dissatisfied with our choice and complain to him later. Michael assured him that the bride wasn't worried about the cake (she was worried about her grades, needlessly, as usual) and outlined the basic requirements: white cake, white frosting, a white couple on top. I don't think the baker appreciated Michael's sense of humor. All Eva had to do was buy her wedding gown. If I hadn't been twenty pounds overweight, I'm sure she would have enlisted me to do that too!

I didn't mind doing all this. I was thrilled that Eva and Michael were getting married. He was the nicest guy I knew. Eva didn't deserve him. I wondered if I'd ever plan my own wedding. I figured this was the closest I'd come. I felt this way despite the fact that for the first time in my life a man was seriously interested in me. Actually, I was seriously interested in him first. It took some time for the feeling to become mutual. I was the one who asked for a date first. I disguised this move by inviting him over for a sumptuous dinner—with my father. I suspected Eric was interested in meeting *him* anyway. But when he kissed me goodnight, I really didn't care. Eric was a graduate student and had been one of my instructors at Mansfield University. He was thirteen years my senior, a foot taller, and very handsome. He could also be quite charming.

As the summer progressed, I found myself more deeply involved in my romance with Eric. I was making up for lost time. Until now, I'd "dated" only two men: Robert, an old high school acquaintance, and Peter, an even older skating buddy. But Bob was a seminarian and Pete was gay, so they didn't really count. My relationship with Eric was thus important for me, personally, as well as for establishing my status as a "normal" twenty-year-old woman. Of course, Eric knew I had lupus. He saw me frequently taking a lot of pills and I simply told him what they were for. It was not a major issue for him. My condition was stable at the time, and neither of us wanted to make a serious commitment. We never considered marriage or children. As for the latter, my only concern was to not get pregnant.

Luckily, I never had to talk about sex or birth control with Dr. Rozen. He retired and I was turned over to Dr. Levine. This change was more welcomed than traumatic. Still, it was another transition, starting from scratch with another doctor. Fortunately, the switch came when my lupus was under control; Dr. Levine was satisfied to continue to monitor my disease while I continued to manage it. His laissez faire attitude immediately endeared him to me.

In a quiet sort of way, Dr. Levine was a very nice person. He was much younger than the other doctors I'd had, closer to my age than my father's, and better looking. Or maybe I was just beginning to notice such things. He was easy to talk to. For him, listening alone was "doing something." I planned to be in town for four more years to finish a PhD; I hoped Dr. Levine's local academic commitments would last as long.

* * *

July 3, 1976, was fast approaching. My twenty-first birthday—officially, an adult. I had been living with lupus for nearly eight years. I had been treated, most of this time, as someone much older than my years. No detail of my disease, no lab result, no potentially harmful side effect of my treatment, was ever hidden from me. There was, however, another very important aspect of living with a chronic illness—perhaps the *only* one—that my father never discussed with me: paying for medical care and, more specifically, obtaining medical insurance.

As a student, I was, in the eyes of the insurance world, still a dependent, covered under my father's medical insurance policy through his employer. This policy paid for all my outpatient laboratory tests and would have paid for any hospitalizations. In addition, because my father was a physician, I was in a somewhat peculiar position when it came to paying for office visits to doctors: Back then, there still prevailed the tradition of "professional courtesy," the practice of physicians waiving charges for services provided to other physicians and their families. I also knew that my father made enough money so that finances were not a problem. I never had to think about where the money came from for food, or the gas in my car, or my tuition at college. My father was by no means frivolous about money, but, in his own way, he was very generous. So why should I worry about medical bills?

Until now, I had concerned myself only with the personal dimension of coping with a chronic illness. It was time for me to learn about coping with its economic dimension. Contrary to popular belief, it is possible to live with a chronic illness *without* facing financial ruin. Actually, managing the financial aspect of illness is almost as important as managing its medical aspect. However, as with any other kind of financial planning, you can't do this if you don't know how. This, too, is something one has to study and learn.

The cost of medical care is a matter of concern for everyone, healthy or ill. For a chronically ill person the expenses are continuous and unremitting and ought to be a paramount consideration. Paradoxically, being chronically ill offers a potential advantage for getting a financial handle on medical problems. While a healthy person may be tempted to ignore the need for medical insurance, a chronically ill person can't afford such idiocy. Unfortunately, physicians rarely if ever discuss the monetary aspects of illness with the patient, probably because they are unable to give patients advice about medical insurance. This is not meant as a criticism. Would anyone consult an architect for homeowner's insurance? Or an automotive engineer for car insurance?

My particular situation—a young adult with a chronic illness and a financially comfortable family—is far from unique. Obviously, I am not in a position to offer advice to the many people who are desperately poor. Nor need I say anything to those who are so wealthy that they don't have to think about money at all. Most people in this country fall somewhere between these extremes. All of us, therefore, have much to learn about health insurance. Many people, however, have as much dread of this subject as they do of illness itself. Worse, they lull themselves into the belief that when things go sour, *someone* will take care of the costs of illness, just as *someone* will take care of the disease.

There are two types of medical insurance: public and private. Public medical insurance, in turn, is of two kinds: Medicaid and Medicare. *Medicaid* is a combined federal and state program, providing medical coverage that varies in amount from state to state. The basic eligibility requirement is low income (as defined by the government). *Medicare* is a federal program of health insurance provided to persons sixty-five or older, or to those disabled, regardless of income. Clearly, most middle-income American adults under sixty-five cannot expect protection from public health insurance programs.

In the private sector for health insurance, the choices are numerous and not necessarily unavailable to the chronically ill. Again, planning ahead is essential. If you are a healthy adult, the chances are that you have a job; and, if you have a job (unless it is a minimum-wage job), that you have medical insurance as part of the benefit package of your employment. Depending on the kind of employer you work for, you may or may not pay the premiums yourself; also, some employers offer several options, with different levels or types of coverage and corresponding ranges in cost. Health insurance is an important benefit associated with employment and should be taken into consideration when looking for a job, especially if you *already have* a chronic illness. Unfortunately, as medical costs continue to rise, employer-provided health insurance will undoubtedly become less extensive and more restrictive. During continuous employment at the same institution from 1980 to 1990, my coverage went from 100 percent with no premium or deductible, to 80 percent with an annually escalating premium and a $200 deductible.

The advantage for the chronically ill employee is that the employer's insurance carrier cannot, under a "group plan," deny coverage to a member of the work force, no matter how unhealthy that particular person might be. Usually, the plan has a "pre-existing condition" clause, excluding coverage for that condition during the first twelve months of the policy. After a year, no exclusion is allowed. Facing a lifetime of expenses, this is not a bad deal. If you are not employed but are a dependent, or are married to someone who has a job, the chances are that you are covered in a similar fashion.

* * *

For the time being, my best bet insurance-wise was either to remain a student, dependent on my father (a status for which the maximum age is twenty-five), or get married and be dependent on a husband. The former status seemed more realistic, even if not more desirable. I had no immediate plans to work (I still thought of studying as legitimate work), so for now I was off the hook. All I needed to know was my father's Blue Cross number. I'd never even *seen* a bill. The outpatient laboratory at Mansfield General sent them directly to the insurance company for payment.

It never occurred to me that the coverage I had was insufficient, or could be improved upon. Wasn't Blue Cross the creme-de-la-creme? Then one day I received some unsolicited literature in the mail. In addition to the honor of being salutatorian of the Class of 1976, I had been awarded membership in two nationally recognized college honor societies: Phi Beta Kappa and Phi Kappa Phi. Almost everything I received from either group concerned requests for money. I usually opened the envelopes directly over the trash can. But this time I received some fliers advertising insurance policies I'd never heard of before.

At first, nothing looked particularly interesting. I already had "group health" insurance under my father's Blue Cross/Blue Shield plan. I didn't need more of that. You had to be employed full time to qualify for "disability insurance." That wasn't for me either. Life insurance I'd never given much thought to. I was young and had no dependents. I also assumed that should I want such insurance I would find it too expensive to make it worthwhile, if not impossible to obtain. I read the flyer more closely. You could purchase a life insurance policy offering the *minimum* benefit ($10,000 in this case) *without* any examination. Moreover, since it was part of a group plan, the annual premium was low, less than the cost of one dinner at a fancy restaurant. I would be foolish to pass this one up. After all, I'd always thought I was likely to die young. I started to fill out the application, as my father studied the remaining flyers. I debated whether to make him, or Eva, the beneficiary.

My father then insisted that I also purchase both the "Excess Major Medical" and "In-Hospital Cash Plan" policies, which were also available without a medical examination. What would I want such insurance for? Were they worth the money? Contrary to popular prejudice, such policies are numerous and widely available, even to chronically ill persons. It is very likely that the person reading this has come across one and has probably thrown it away. In my experience, hardly a month goes by when I don't receive such an unsolicited offer in the mail. Some come directly from insurance carriers, others from major credit card companies, still others from nationwide department store chains. Regardless of the source, these policies offer coverage at a group rate and provide automatic coverage, except for a waiting period for pre-existing conditions.

There are important differences between excess major medical and hospital cash plans. Hospital cash plans are simpler. They pay, directly to the insured, a set amount for each day spent in the hospital—the sum typically varying from $30 to $100 per day. The premiums vary accordingly, usually from $125 to $250 per year for a person under the age of thirty-five. (They are slightly higher for the next age bracket.) The benefit money goes directly to patient, not to the hospital or the doctors, regardless of any other insurance coverage the person may have. However, the premiums are not insignificant. And you must end up in the hospital to reap the "benefits."

I didn't much like the sound of it. It was a depressing prospect. In the case of life insurance, the money at least went to a beneficiary who might make good use of it. But what good would money be to me for being hospitalized? If I could stay well enough to avoid hospitalization, as I had for nearly a decade, the premiums were a huge waste. And if I became so ill as to require hospitalization, surely I would never survive the ordeal to enjoy the rewards.

As it turned out, I was wrong on all counts. I was too morbid, too fatalistic, too cheap, and too naive. Although good doctors, good fortune, and a good father had spared me, thus far, from having to be hospitalized, the chances of my lupus eventually necessitating such a sojourn were very high indeed. If ever there was a sound financial gamble, however perverse, *this was it*. My father forced me to act like an adult, even if he did order me around like a daughter.

The excess major medical policy appealed to me even less. I read and re-read the description, and was convinced it duplicated my Blue Cross/Blue Shield coverage. In any case, it was virtually impossible to understand what "excess" meant. The policy began with a confusing statement concerning a *fifteen thousand dollar* deductible. My father explained that this meant $15,000 in medical expenses had to be incurred in a year before any benefits would be paid, not that the $15,000 had to come out of my own (or his) pocket. For example, if I was in the hospital for a month, or even less, I'd incur that much or more—most, if not all, paid by Blue Cross. So far I followed the accounting. The excess major medical policy would then cover what Blue Cross did not. I still couldn't understand *what*. The cost of this policy, however, was low, less than fifty dollars a year—and not worth arguing about. Or as my father liked to say, "Less than you spend on one skirt." If he only knew how much I spend today.

Much as I wanted to be autonomous, I was growing weary of plodding through insurance policies, never mind discussing with my father the statistical probabilities of my becoming sick enough to "benefit" from them. I filled out the forms, wrote out the checks for the first installment on the premiums, and put them in the mail. Enough of this. Surely this was no way to make money.

In a few weeks, the policies arrived. I filed them away in my highly organized style and forgot about them. So did my father. Completely.

* * *

After a summer of excitement and relaxation—Eva's wedding, Eric-in-my-life, and a part-time job typing Family Court transcripts—I started graduate school in September 1976. Actually, I wasn't too keen about this project of getting a PhD in philosophy, but it seemed like the only logical thing to do. I had a Weaver Fellowship, and the people in the philosophy department at Mansfield University were begging me to join their program. This time it wasn't the stress that got to me; instead, it was the pretentious pseudointellectual atmosphere of the whole enterprise. After several weeks debating whether the blackboard in the classroom was real or not, I quit. Just plain quit, like a bored healthy student. No excuses this time.

While taking a break from academia, I decided to get a real job. My father wasn't very happy about my decision. He thought I was throwing away *two* attractive fellowships. Neither was Eric. He held out more promise for my future as a scholar than he did for his own. I was distressed too. I didn't want to disappoint the two most important men in my life.

I quickly landed a job at one of the local television stations. It wasn't anything glamorous. I was a "traffic clerk"—and took home less than $100 a week. But now I had my own Blue Cross card! It saddened me that I got the job largely on the basis of my typing skills. This is where all that "therapeutic typing" of John Stuart Mill had gotten me.

However, the job served a good purpose. It gave me a breathing spell. I could step away from the academic world and think about what I really wanted to do. And, at long last, it allowed me to slow down, to stop the wild rush I had been in to move on. In my race against myself to "not waste time," I finally paused: I was still only *twenty-one years old*. Most people my age hadn't graduated from college yet.

In the meantime, I had to adjust to *another* new doctor. Dr. Levine left town, and academic medicine, to open a private practice in another city. I guess he got fed up with academia, too! By now I was sure I would never find another doctor as devoted as Dr. Patterson, so it was best to stop hoping. I entered into yet another physician relationship with an open mind. Dr. Crane was a rheumatologist at Mansfield General, a colleague of Dr. Levine's. Like Dr. Levine, he was relatively young. Reserved, yet friendly. I had always felt relaxed with physicians; now I was beginning to learn how to make *them* feel relaxed as well.

My job at the television station didn't lead to celebrity status on the six o'clock evening news. In fact, it was so mindless that after a few months I felt I needed some other activity to fill out my day. Mansfield University offered evening classes. By sheer accident, I ran into a friend of Eva's from MacArthur High. Three years older than me, Sarah had just returned home—overeducated and unemployed. She had decided to turn her unmarketable degrees in music into something practical by going for a master's degree in library science. She was ready to begin school in a week and suggested I join her.

"LIBRARY SCHOOL?" What the hell, I thought. And for the time being, I could also keep my job. No sudden, drastic move this time.

* * *

During my brief career in television I stumbled on an organization I'd never come across before: the Lupus Foundation of America. The station had recently made a public service announcement about lupus that went on to win an award. It was my job to schedule announcements such as these during times when no commercial time had been sold, which usually meant at one o'clock in the morning when hardly anyone saw them.

I wondered whether I should attend one of the group's monthly meetings. After putting it off a few times, I decided I had nothing to lose. While I have no desire to disparage the importance of such support groups, *I* found the experience more than merely a waste of a good Sunday afternoon. Instead of being enlightening or uplifting, the meeting was depressing and demeaning.

I might have been willing to overlook the simplicity of the "message" had it been delivered in a more existentially attractive context. To be sure, we were all gathered together because we shared a common misfortune. Maybe we might also share some common horror stories—about the illness, experiences with doctors, discrimination at work or at school. But, after all, our common bond—our experiences as lupus patients—was supposed to *support* us, not undermine our self-confidence. No one talked about anything other than being ill. Life seemed filled with nothing but disappointment and despair, which the group, as a formal gathering, seemed intent on legitimizing as both involuntary and insurmountable. Discussion centered on our need for other peoples' attention and sympathy; nothing was said about our responsibility and scope for control. The group did not see, let alone want to discuss, the affliction as an adversity to overcome; instead, it was completely overcome by the adversity of the affliction itself. In the end, I had very little in common with the members of this group because, as Nietzsche remarked, "Shared joys make a friend, not shared sufferings." I never went back.

Since then I have found other groups more helpful. For example, the national (or "parent") chapter of the Lupus Foundation of America is a good source of information on the latest advances in research as well as on related subjects such as health insurance and Social Security. The organization publishes an excellent newsletter, *Lupus News*. Years later, I joined a local chapter of the Arthritis Foundation. This group, made up largely of people over the age of fifty, gets together several times a week—not so members can wallow in their woes, but to engage in aquatic exercises and swim. Those not up to working out on a particular day often come along anyway, to sit by the pool and cheer the others on instead of sitting at home alone, feeling miserable.

* * *

Six months at the television station made the alternative of life as a librarian look a whole lot more attractive. I applied for and received a scholarship to finish my master's in library science, quit my job, and resumed my former life as a full-time student. No sooner was I back on the academic stage than I fell right back into my old role of superachieving. I began to reconsider pursuing the PhD I had sworn I'd put out of my mind for good. This time, I convinced myself that I was being more practical—and I was. An advanced degree in an academic subject would, together with my library degree, greatly enhance my job prospects as a librarian. This was reasonable. Next I talked myself into believing that to gain intellectually from the experience I should continue my graduate work at another institution, one with a "suitable" program in political philosophy. There was no such offering at Mansfield University. I had tried, unsuccessfully, to adapt my interests to the more conventional curriculum of its philosophy department. I could, at least temporarily, convince myself of anything.

In addition to another shot at a PhD, I was also forcing myself into another shot at living away from home. I thought I would probably have to do this sooner or later anyway. In selecting a graduate school I used two criteria besides the academic curriculum: medical and economic. I had to go somewhere near decent medical facilities, and I wanted a scholarship. I was escalating my requirements so high I wondered if I wasn't really trying to guarantee I wouldn't find such a place and could stay at home with a good conscience.

No such luck. I found the perfect school, got a research assistantship and a medical referral, and prepared for my departure. It had been six years since I had tried to leave home the first time. I couldn't sit back any longer. As I packed my books, I came across a copy of Seneca's *Works* and noticed an appropriately underlined passage: "If a man is to know himself, he must be tested. No one knows what he can accomplish except by trying."

* * *

The place I chose was a large university located in Asheville, a small southern city. It has a well-known teaching hospital affiliated with it, and it was a very long day's drive from my home in Mansfield.

A month before moving south, in late August 1978, my father and I went to Asheville and explored the city together. I rented a nice one-bedroom furnished apartment close to the university. I knew I was better suited to living alone and being lonely than to sharing an apartment with a stranger. At first, I was more than a little miserable. Older and wiser, this time I *knew* I was just homesick. Why shouldn't I miss being home? I lived in a nice, big house; I got along extremely well with the only other occupant, my father; I could come and go, more or less, as I pleased; I had good friends in Mansfield; and Eric was still in my life—there. One would have to be crazy *not* to miss all that.

After scheduling my classes for the semester, I scheduled my first medical appointment—with Dr. Gould, a rheumatologist, and Dr. Laughton, one of his "fellows." To my pleasant surprise and pleasure, *this* teaching hospital had a group of "private clinics," located in a row of separate buildings on a tree-lined street adjacent to the main campus of the university. No massive hospital building, no parking garage, no bodies on stretchers! The Arthritis Clinic was located on one floor of an attractive, nineteenth-century red brick house only a block from the library. It was more like going to another class than to a doctor's office. One day a week the operation of the Arthritis Clinic was devoted entirely to seeing patients with lupus.

I sat in the waiting room reading Aristotle's *Politics*. It was as quiet and comfortable as in the library. I hardly noticed the time until my name was called. I was aware of the many people waiting and of the fact that quite a few did not fit the "you-don't-look-like-there's-anything-wrong-with-you" image. In fact, it was obvious that many were gravely ill. Dr. Gould and Dr. Laughton greeted me politely and asked me to come into their office. Another pleasant surprise: They would take my "history" while I remained seated, fully dressed.

My experiences at the Lupus Clinic in Asheville were different in several important respects from any medical encounters I had faced to date. In the first place, I was completely on my own. My father, Dr. Hauser (the doctor I'd known the longest and who knew me best), and Dr. Crane (the latest member of my medical entourage, who was moving at the same time anyway) were hundreds of miles away. What of all those years, at home, when I claimed to possess so much autonomy and responsibility? It was true. But now I saw it in a different light. For better or worse—and usually for better—my father had, from the very beginning of my illness, played a crucial role in the planning of my health care. In a way, he was like an athletic coach, training me to play the game. He rarely came right out onto the field, but he was always there on the sidelines, signalling, sometimes even yelling. He was also a team manager, helping select the other players. And, admittedly, all the players—my *doctors* no less than me—knew who called a lot of the plays. So while I always had the ultimate authority over particular decisions regarding my medical treatment, I can scarcely recall doing so without at least talking it over with my father. I had no reason not to. Similarly, while all my doctors in Mansfield had treated me with the utmost sense of respect and responsibility (even when I was a teenager), they too usually consulted, or at least communicated, with my father. This did not mean that they—or my father—ever went behind my back. Last, but not least, my father was in an unusual, though not unique, position to offer both professional and personal guidance: professional, based on his knowledge as a physician, which had already proved remarkable (especially for a psychiatrist); personal, based on his dual role as parent and colleague.

Now I was away from home field, playing with new players, and no local manager. Of course, I still kept in touch with the coach by telephone. But the other players didn't. None of the doctors at the Lupus Clinic knew my father personally, although they knew "of" him professionally—all too well I sometimes felt—from his writings. They had no way of knowing of his past propinquity to me or my previous physicians. I was on my own.

Dr. Gould and Dr. Laughton had long reports from Dr. Hauser and Dr. Crane recounting the significant events of my medical odyssey, but they wanted me to recount the story in my own words. They knew what had taken place and when, but they wanted me to explain *why* I was given such-and-such medication or *why* I had *not* undergone such-and-such a test.

My new doctors agreed to continue with my established regimen: the same drugs (Prednisone and Imuran) in the same doses (now "only" 10 and 50 milligrams a day, respectively); the same routine of blood tests, urinalyses, and accounts of my day-to-day activities. Despite their heavy research interests, Dr. Gould and Dr. Laughton showed concern for the patient as a person, not just as a carrier of lupus. One day, however, the conversation with Dr. Laughton broached a new subject, and the first sign of tension.

"Suzy, how come you never had a kidney biopsy, prior to the diagnosis of SLE, or any time since then?"

This question didn't come as a total surprise. Shortly before I left Mansfield, during my last appointment with him, Dr. Crane briefed me about what to expect in Asheville. Among the things he told me—warned me might be more appropriate—was that the doctors were very interested in lupus research. Now I remembered Dr. Crane's parting words of advice: "If it were *my* kidney, I'd leave it alone." Those were his very words and, as I sat there, they rang in my head loud and clear.

"Well, Dr. Laughton, there are many reasons. When I first became ill, late in 1968, my father felt it was risky. My doctor at the time concurred. When the question came up again a few months later, there was no need for it, as there was enough evidence, both from my clinical manifestations and from my laboratory results, to determine a proper diagnosis and course of treatment. That has continued to be the case over the years. The results of a kidney biopsy would not have altered the course of treatment, so it has always seemed to be an unnecessary risk—with no possible benefit."

At the time (1977), *The Merck Manual* stated,

> Kidney biopsy is unnecessary unless the diagnosis is uncertain. Biopsy may be helpful late in the course of renal disease to determine whether medi-

cal therapy should be continued or whether dialysis and transplantation should be considered.

It was not until the next edition, printed in 1982, that the following revealing sentence was inserted between the two above: "Although the findings on biopsy are of academic interest, there is usually a good response to treatment regardless of the findings." The business of a kidney biopsy never came up again.

The research interests of the doctors at the Lupus Clinic were not limited to the biological dimension of the disease. They were interested in its psychiatric aspects as well. For the physician, this is a happy hunting ground indeed; for the patient, it can be a no-win situation. If you, the patient, are too concerned about your illness, you are obsessed, maybe depressed as well; if you seem to be coping too well, you are denying your illness. I recalled an old joke my father was fond of recounting about psychoanalysis, whose butt is the analyst who can find sickness in whatever the patient does: "If the patient is early for his appointment, he is anxious; if he is late, he is hostile; and if he is on time, he is compulsive."

So I was prepared for this, too—although it occurred to me that, given who I was, they might steer clear of this subject. Maybe they were just testing me—to see if I were a true SZASZ. I soon discovered what I suspected all along: namely, that the more interested doctors are in doing something *for* you, the more likely they'll want to do something *to* you. However, just as I had viewed having my kidney probed with a needle as needless, so I viewed having my mind probed verbally as equally unwarranted and intrusive.

One day in mid-December the absurdity of this sort of interrogation reached a new height. Facing the pressures of four final examinations and two major term papers, I nonetheless kept my monthly appointment with Dr. Laughton. I was growing to like, and appreciate, my relationship with him and realized it was enhanced by regular meetings. I never minded our disagreements. I enjoyed "debating" and Dr. Laughton was always thoughtful and unhurried. But sometimes he did take himself a little too seriously.

I was accustomed to his asking, "Suzy, are you experiencing any unusual anxiety or tension in your life right now?" On this day I didn't refrain from blurting out the first words that came to my mind: "Don't you know what time of year it is? Of course I'm anxious and tense! How did *you* feel the week before national boards?"

Dr. Laughton didn't take my remarks exactly the way I intended. But he never again discussed my personal life—unless *I* initiated the dialogue.

I *was* capable of handling the medical scene on my own: no invasive diagnostic tests, no psychobabble. I respected my doctors, as long as they respected my wishes.

Seven

To be nobody-but-myself—in a world which is doing its best, night and day, to make you everybody else—means to fight the hardest battle which any human being can fight, and never stop fighting.
—e e cummings

I returned to Asheville after Christmas vacation to the South's worst winter in a century and to the news of having gotten straight "A's" in the four courses I had just completed. I had always had the drive to get good grades. But these grades had practical importance, as the fellowships awarded for the second year of graduate school depended entirely on the first semester's performance. So, everything was going well, better than I had hoped. On top of my good grades and a much-coveted research assistantship, I was asked to serve as a teaching assistant for an introductory course in political theory—the first time a *first-year* graduate student had ever been asked to do so. All this recognition began to go to my head, making me think again about a career as a professor instead of as a librarian. I soon returned to my senses.

On my way to class one cold morning I slipped on a patch of ice and landed hard on my coccyx. After a few moments to catch my breath I got up and drove off to school. I hoped a lively seminar might distract me from my pain. But, try as I might, I couldn't concentrate. Instead of joining in the discussion on "social contract" theories, I began to contemplate where my life was going. I enjoyed the reading. I enjoyed the writing. I enjoyed debating with my colleagues. But what was it all *for*? How would I feel once I got through with school, had my PhD, and was a professor? Would leading such discussions as the teacher be any more satisfying than participating in them as a student? Would publishing essays in scholarly journals be any more rewarding than getting another "A" on a term paper? Was this any way to live—or make a living?

Besides, I already had a marketable skill: my master's degree in library science. Moreover, I had been working for my advisor as his research assistant, in effect as his private, part-time librarian! I enjoyed ferreting out obscure references and compiling bibliographies—more than my own studies. Maybe a library *job* was the perfect combination of scholarship and practicality: the seriousness of academia without the pretension. I decided to quit graduate school and look for an academic library position.

I resolved, however, to continue in school while looking for a job. No more bridge-burning. Although the job market for librarians was much better than for PhDs in political theory, I did not expect to get a job offer until the beginning of the next academic year, nearly six months away. I could complete the coursework for my master's, write my thesis later, and eventually get another degree—and a job.

I scoured library journals for job postings and composed a résumé. I had a part-time position as a research assistant, a superior academic background, but no formal library experience. I said not a word about my illness. I was glad that it was "invisible." Of course, it occurred to me that the state of my health might come up during an interview. I knew I wasn't *supposed* to be asked such questions, but what really happened *in practice*?

People in personnel have more subtle methods of interrogation, focusing on gaps of time in your résumé, between jobs or between periods spent in school. I felt some vindication for all my seemingly hasty moves in recent years—there were no noticeable gaps in *my* résumé.

*   *   *

After less than two months of interviewing, I got a job. It was a very good job, indeed: reference librarian at an outstanding university. I would be working with the public, which appealed to my gregarious instincts; I would be giving classes on library research methods to students, which would satisfy my desire to teach; I would be at an Ivy League school, which appealed to my lingering academic snobbery; and I would be only an hour's drive from "home," which meant I could reap the benefits of my close bond with my father, see more of Eric, and still live an independent, socially acceptable adult existence. The only fly in this otherwise fine ointment was that my job search was completed much sooner than I expected. I had to report to work in May. I couldn't complete the coursework for the spring semester, much less make any significant headway on my thesis. Since my new employer didn't show much interest in my finishing the second master's degree, I didn't agonize over it either. I submitted requests for "incompletes" and met one last time with my advisor who, instead of chastising me for abandoning what everyone said was a promising career as a political theorist, commended me for the work I had done and congratulated me on my decision and new appointment. My peers seemed equally enthusiastic, perhaps because with me gone, one research assistantship and one teaching assistantship were up for grabs.

I had one more appointment with Dr. Laughton before leaving Asheville. I think we were both a little sorry that this was our last meeting. Despite occasional disagreements, we had established a very decent doctor-patient relationship. I participated in his research studies, even if I didn't go along with all his requests. And he explained many tests and procedures to me, in greater detail than any doctor before. In seven months, Dr. Laughton did not propose a single change in my treatment. Until today.

Months earlier, Dr. Laughton had expressed concern over my taking Imuran. I had been on the drug for nearly six years, primarily for its steroid-sparing effect. During this time I had, indeed, managed to reduce my Prednisone dosage from a high of 125 milligrams every other day to 10 milligrams every day. But it didn't look as if I could ever manage on less than that, or that I would ever get off the steroids entirely. While I was on a relatively low dose, I was nonetheless "dependent," no longer able to maintain an alternate-day regimen. As far as Dr. Laughton was concerned, I was subjecting myself to the long-term ill effects of two drugs, one of which—Imuran, a known carcinogen—I probably didn't need. Its risks seemed to outweigh its benefits. This made sense, but I decided to postpone acting on Dr. Laughton's recommendation to discontinue the Imuran. I didn't want to make a major change in the management of my disease at a time rife with personal change as well.

I left the Lupus Clinic with Dr. Laughton's written summary of my case, not knowing who would be its next recipient. Perhaps because of the added burden of packing and the anticipation of moving, the results of my last visit to the laboratory showed increased signs of disease activity. Most notably, my complement had dropped significantly. "Complement" was one of those tests I'd learned a lot about from Dr. Laughton. The antigen-antibody system—which both fights infection and mediates autoimmune diseases—comprises over two dozen forms of complement, that is, blood proteins. Although the normal total complement is between 50 and 100, depending on the laboratory, mine was never higher than 40. Now it was down to 15. In addition, my increased sed rate also indicated renewed disease activity. Lastly, my ANA (anti-nuclear antibody test) was at a higher titer than usual, out of even *my* range of abnormal. I re-read Dr. Laughton's words and numbers with some anxiety. "Thus, although Ms. Szasz has shown essentially no clinical activity except for some occasional fatigue and minimal arthralgias, she has started to show some serological activity and will need closer scrutiny."

* * *

It didn't take me long to find a charming apartment in the small town of Concord. Like the apartment I had in Asheville, this one was so close to campus even I could walk to work when the sun wasn't shining (which is most of the time around here), or could take a short bus ride if I wanted to save my energy. I decided not to apply for a special parking permit, at least for now. When possible, I still tried to pass as "normal."

It took even less time for me to feel back at "home." I was only fifty miles from my father's house in Thornden, a suburb of Mansfield he'd moved to several years before. I could visit whenever I wanted without taking time off from work. Also, I was still "seeing" Eric. I didn't know where our relationship was going, if anywhere, but I enjoyed his company—and, of course, the fact that it made me more socially acceptable. I was amazed at how atypical it was to be a single, unattached female. In Concord, it often seemed more deviant to be single and heterosexual than to be gay.

Settling into a new medical arrangement was not as easy as finding a job and an apartment. Fortunately, Dr. Hauser was still monitoring my case, however minimally, and he still had connections. But he was getting older and his health was deteriorating. Unlike in earlier times, he was now at a loss about whom to recommend for me. He was always candid and critical with me, just like my father. "I wouldn't send my *dog* to that one," was his remark about several potential candidates.

I decided I had nothing to lose by exploring the possibilities of finding a physician in Concord. With Mansfield General only an hour's drive away, the town offered no booming medical community. But as my father loved to say in such dilemmas, "You only need *one*." Fortunately, Dr. Laughton's alarm concerning the serological activity of my lupus proved to be false. Dr. Hauser ordered another series of laboratory tests, and while the results were not normal—mine never were—they were less startling.

I concluded that the new arrangement I was about to make with a local physician was, though not ideal, probably workable. Dr. Cohen, a rheumatologist, had an office conveniently located right on campus. He also had access to the laboratory facilities at Concord Community Hospital. Moreover, Dr. Hauser "knew of" Dr. Cohen and had no objections to the choice, which was virtually an endorsement. Dr. Cohen, who had no special interest in lupus, was relaxed, easy to talk to, and happy to leave things as they were, all of which suited me just fine.

The repeated changes of doctors made me realize that I was the only constant when it came to managing my condition. During these first few months in Concord, I became very aware of the dilemma of when-to-call/when-not-to-call a doctor: If you don't call, you might be ignoring something serious; if you call every time you notice something unusual, your complaints may be interpreted as pleas for intervention, which may be unnecessary or harmful. As things turned out, it was totally impossible to reach Dr. Cohen when one needed him. Once I waited two days for a response to a particular query. On the third day, I was no worse and concluded that my call, at least this time, had been unnecessary. But I also realized that one day I might need more help. Unless I had a physician ready and willing to listen, and act accordingly, a minor problem could become major. It was clear that the arrangement with Dr. Cohen could not last long.

* * *

My job at the library was great, but I had never worked so hard in my life. School never presented so demanding a physical schedule. I had been told about the importance of getting adequate rest for years. For me, this was critical to lessen the possibility of having a lupus "flare." As a student, finding the time to rest had never been a problem. Now, with less of my time under my own control, I became more aware of what little free time I had left outside of work.

In October 1979 I received my first six-month performance evaluation at the library. It was glowing. The report from the laboratory following my last appointment with the gynecologist was less encouraging.

I'd been seeing Dr. Klein for more than a decade, and hadn't had any problems since the bleeding episode that heralded the onset of my lupus. But after a routine six-month examination, Dr. Klein called to say that my Pap smear was slightly abnormal, showing cervical dysplasia. His advice was conservative—repeat the test every three months—but the warning flag was hoisted: The dysplasia (abnormal growth of cells) could be an early sign of cervical cancer, possibly brought on by all those years of taking Imuran.

But as yet no one seemed alarmed: not Dr. Klein, not Dr. Hauser, not my father (who gets nervous about my health at the slightest provocation), not myself, and certainly not Dr. Cohen, who wouldn't even hear the news until my next appointment with him. That was four months away. There was no point in calling him before then. I could wait until I had the results of a second Pap smear to report. We could discuss discontinuing the Imuran then too. I didn't think that required immediate attention either, based on the evidence of only one slightly abnormal test. I was, of course, also trying to dismiss the suspicion Dr. Laughton had raised months before.

At the end of the next three months my dysplasia worsened. Dr. Klein wanted me off the Imuran, Dr. Hauser concurred, and Dr. Cohen had no opinion. I was uneasy about what effect discontinuing the Imuran might have on my lupus. But the prospect of cervical cancer was more immediate and more disturbing. In January of 1980 I stopped taking Imuran, had another Pap smear, and a cervical punch biopsy. With three consecutive abnormal reports in hand, Dr. Klein recommended I undergo a cervical cone biopsy. After eleven years of living with lupus as an outpatient, I would finally have to accept being hospitalized.

The date of the operation was set for late June. The semester would be over, the library would be quiet, and I wouldn't feel too guilty about being away from work for a few weeks.

* * *

Eric and I had been seeing each other—a wonderfully vacuous expression that happens to capture the character of our relationship all too well—since my graduation from college. Four years.

Memorial Day 1980 was an unusually warm weekend for the Northeast. I drove up Friday evening from Concord to Eric's apartment in Mansfield and we decided to head for the Adirondack Mountains the next morning. We didn't know exactly where we were going; that was part of the fun of it. It was the first time the two of us had gone away together. I didn't care where we went.

By Saturday afternoon, we were in the mountains. We drove on, stopping at Blue Mountain Lake. It was early evening by now, sufficiently late, I thought, to be "sun safe" for a motorboat ride on the lake. It was also cool enough to put on a long-sleeve jacket. With blue jeans, hat on my head, and a fresh layer of "Number 15" over any remaining exposed skin, I felt I was being careful enough. Actually, it was getting so late that the man at the rental boat dock was about to close up shop. Eric jumped out of the car and ran ahead to catch his attention. He must have told the guy I had only six months to live, because when I caught up with them the man had decided to stick around so we could go out on the lake for half an hour. He looked at me with a combination of disbelief and sorrow as he handed Eric the keys to the boat.

The half hour ended much too quickly. The lake was crystal clear, the sunset spectacular. Okay, it was all very romantic. What we didn't count on were the black flies, notorious in the area at this time of year. These were no ordinary flies: They were monsters! We were both bitten up good.

By next morning, the black flies were forgotten, while the loveliness of the evening lingered. We drove on—up the west side of Lake Champlain, nearly to the Canadian border; down the east side through Vermont; into the Berkshire Mountains of western Massachusetts. There we would stop and surprise Eric's parents with a brief visit, spend the night, and return to Mansfield on Monday.

It was a glorious weekend. The weather held up, the car held up, our relationship held up. When I returned to my apartment, late Monday night, my only regret was that we hadn't been able to stay away a few days longer. I undressed for bed, looked at my body in the mirror, and froze in fear and horror: My chest was covered with a rash so repulsive it defies description. I turned off the lights and went to bed.

The six-thirty a.m. alarm startled me. I went to the mirror to inspect the rash. It was no worse, but also no better. I decided to "wait and see" before calling the doctor. I didn't even call my father. Typically, I would tell him about anything that disturbed me, medical or otherwise; but this seemed too disgusting to talk about with anyone, except maybe Eric, since he'd been bitten up too. I dressed for work, in the loosest-fitting garment I could find so as not to irritate the lesions. The rash was sore and itchy and it worried me. I didn't know what to do. I only knew I didn't want anyone to see my chest the way it looked. I decided to wait until Friday afternoon, after work, then drive to Mansfield for the weekend. What I hoped to accomplish there I didn't know.

By Friday, my skin looked worse. Much worse. As I pondered my predicament, it dawned on me that Eva and Michael were coming home for a visit. Until a year ago, they had lived nearby while attending medical school and visited frequently on weekends. When I returned to the Northeast, they moved to the West Coast for their residencies. Since Eva and I tended to (quietly) compete for my father's attentions, and I had so much more contact with him than my sister, I thought I'd be nice and make myself scarce for their arrival by spending Friday night with Eric. There would be plenty of time for a family reunion later.

Eric and I spent a tense evening together. For obvious reasons, he didn't want to get near me. I could understand that, but it hurt just the same. Perhaps he also felt somewhat responsible for my condition, and didn't want to be reminded of it. I needed emotional support, and I wasn't getting any. It occurred to me that this was the first time in four years that Eric had actually seen me *sick*. I sensed, all too clearly from this seemingly minor incident, that he would never be able to see me through a serious lupus flare.

When I awoke Saturday morning, I didn't even need to look in the mirror. There were several huge blisters, like those that follow a burn, *on my hands too*. My silence and my hiding were over, that much was clear. I left Eric's apartment and went "home."

I decided to consult Eva first. After all, she was my sister. She was also a physician, by this time a second-year resident in pediatrics. Her first reaction, appropriately enough, was that of a sister, not a doctor.

"God, that is GROOOSS!!" She was shocked and repelled. After carefully performing a physical examination, she informed me, in no uncertain terms, that something *had* to be done, now. Then, reverting to her role as the big sister, she yelled out from one of the upstairs bedrooms at my father's house where we were holding our private medical consultation, "DADDY!!! COME HERE QUICK!!!"

No doubt assuming we were just screaming at each other as we often did, with one of us calling for intervention, my father didn't immediately respond. He had learned to let us battle things out ourselves. After another shriek, he appeared.

One look at his daughters, and my father could tell that we hadn't been fighting. Eva looked at me with her inimitable glare that could be so eloquent. "You'd better tell him—and show him!" I did. Although I was embarrassed by the sight of the lesions, I was not prudish when it came to serious medical matters. This *was* serious. There was no longer any doubt about that. So my father, the physician, took a look. His facial reaction was like Eva's, but his verbal response was more considered and composed.

"I'm going to call Dr. Hauser."

Why hadn't I thought of that? Dr. Hauser was always the doctor to call when we didn't know whom else to call. Not that he would be able to do anything himself, but he would know someone who could. Within the hour, Dr. Hauser called back, having made arrangements for me to see a dermatologist at Mansfield General—Dr. Steiner—*immediately*. Dr. Steiner would meet us at the hospital as soon as we could get there.

The remaining hours of that Saturday afternoon are a blur: Not because I can't remember all that happened, but because so much happened so fast. As I got dressed, Eva volunteered a diagnosis: lupus panniculitis. It was a form of lupus erythematosus in which "non-tender firm nodules . . . occur in the panniculus adiposis [the layer of fat underlying the skin], usually beneath relatively normal appearing skin. Infrequently, the lesions may ulcerate. Systemic involvement is common."* Like my father, who years earlier was eager to offer his medical opinion about my condition, Eva shared his penchant for straying outside her own medical specialty. Along with her diagnosis came a prognosis.

"It's almost always fatal. You have two weeks."

This was a morbid combination of Eva at her worst—the humorist joking around plus the pessimistic doctor. She wanted to come with me to see Dr. Steiner, which was okay with me. That my father would come along too went without saying, for my own moral support and to calm *him* down. My brother-in-law, Michael, had the good sense to stay out of all this and went to play golf.

The drive to the hospital was short and solemn. The atmosphere inside the building was eerie. It was Saturday, mid-afternoon. The clinics and offices were closed for the weekend. There was hardly a soul in sight. The bleak and empty surroundings resonated with Eva's grim diagnosis. We were all familiar with the building and had no difficulty finding Dr. Steiner's office, despite its location in a remote research wing of the hospital.

I don't know what I was expecting, but Sydney Steiner was surely not it. He was very young (I guessed mid-thirties), very tall (not only from my perspective), and very boisterous. His imposing height was perhaps all the more apparent in the presence of not one, but three short people. And he didn't look like a doctor: cut-off shorts, tee-shirt, and an immense beard. Of course, it *was* Saturday afternoon, and he wasn't supposed to have been "working."

After what struck me as a pretty cursory examination—in public, with Eva and my father sitting right there—Dr. Steiner cracked a couple of jokes and, as if he had just examined a corpse, he turned to Eva.:

"So, what do *you* think?"

"Looks like lupus panniculitis."

I was too dumbfounded to say anything. I could only think, "Excuse me? Remember me?" But Eva always did attract men's attentions.

"Bullous impetigo," Dr. Steiner announced calmly. He was firm, but utterly without pomposity. "You must see a lot of that with all the kids you treat!"

"Bullous" is the technical term for blisters filled with fluid. "Impeti-

---

Dorland's Illustrated Medical Dictionary, 26th edition. (Saunders, 1981), p. 958.

go" is an acute inflammatory skin disease usually caused by streptococci or staphylococci bacteria. It is common in children. At least I'd heard of this disease, and knew roughly what it was. Dr. Steiner seemed to find the whole affair rather amusing. He obviously enjoyed teasing my sister for missing such an ordinary diagnosis and me for getting a "kid's disease." Although Dr. Steiner was kind and anything but paternalistic, he made me feel unimportant, if not silly. It was not a case of love at first sight.

Thanks to Dr. Hauser, Dr. Steiner knew I had lupus. So, however ordinary impetigo might be, the lupus made it anything but simple to treat. But Dr. Steiner's confidence was undaunted; he knew exactly how to treat what ailed me. He prescribed 80 milligrams of Prednisone a day—eight times my "normal" regimen!—plus two grams of Dicloxicillin, double the typical dose of a powerful antibiotic. While the steroids might interfere with combating the infection, the infection itself created an unusual stress on the body, requiring more steroids to avoid a lupus flare. As if the ugly blisters weren't worrisome enough, now I was also concerned that the increased Prednisone dosage would turn my face into a balloon and my body into a butterball. Luckily, the antibiotic killed my appetite.

Although he barely spoke a word to me directly, Dr. Steiner did assure me that I could expect to see an improvement in the skin lesions within thirty-six to forty-eight hours. I was to return to his office Monday morning for a complete laboratory workup.

So I had an official diagnosis for what had previously been only something gross and disgusting. But I felt no better. Actually, I soon felt worse—from the nausea and diarrhea brought on by the antibiotic. I spent the rest of the weekend trying to make the most of Eva and Michael's visit. Eva told Eric to stay home and wash everything I'd touched. Sunday evening came, and the rash didn't look any better. Maybe Dr. Steiner was wrong. Maybe it wasn't impetigo after all.

Whatever I had, it was clear I wouldn't be back at the library on Monday morning. I called Jean, my supervisor, and told her not to expect me back the entire week. I tried to sound convincing when I told her there was nothing to worry about. Just some routine tests.

After three days on Dicloxicillin, my skin looked the same. Drama: Ugly Bullae. Act Two: Dr. Steiner, Eva, and my father hovering over me once again. With his confidence a little shaken, Dr. Steiner didn't laugh at the newest opinion, this time offered by my father, who wasn't going to be outdone by these two youngsters: pemphigus, another deadly skin disease, also characterized by bullae without, however, any bacterial infection. The lack of response to the antibiotics supported the diagnosis of this rare and usually fatal disease. I was beginning to think members of my own family could only come up with diagnoses that gave me two weeks to live.

I realized that the possibility of pemphigus was being seriously considered when Dr. Steiner said he wanted to perform a biopsy of the skin lesions. This was obviously the best way to arrive at a correct diagnosis. And, unlike a kidney biopsy, it was perfectly safe. In addition, a culture of the fluid in the blisters would establish the presence or absence of bacteria. The procedure was simple and painless. The worst part was the waiting. The specimen was sent to an out-of-town laboratory. In the meantime, still clinging to his original opinion, Dr. Steiner prescribed a different antibiotic: Erythromycin. Everyone seemed to be grasping at straws.

It slowly dawned on me that not only had I let Dr. Steiner take over my case, I was actually beginning to like the man. I almost hated to admit it. At first, his brashness and *very* casual demeanor turned me off. He didn't seem to be serious, or *act* serious—about anything. Somewhat to my surprise, he didn't hesitate to admit he might be wrong. Moreover, he really did listen to me as easily as he spoke his own mind. It didn't take me long to change my style, too. I found myself acting more relaxed and jocular than I had with any other doctor.

With the biopsy done, Dr. Steiner peered over me, lying on the examination table half-naked, and announced he wanted to take pictures of my lesions for his research. "No DAMNED pictures, Syd!" I exclaimed. I'd never called one of my doctors by his first name before, much less used words like "damned," even humorously.

I went "home," to my father's house in Thornden, and waited. We all waited. Eva and Michael's presence added to the suspense. We waited for the laboratory report on the possibility of pemphigus; for the culture on the presence of staph or strep or nothing; for the effect of the Erythromycin; for the results of the status of my lupus activity. My father's quiet nervousness finally erupted—as did his forehead, with the predictable red rash—only to engage Eva in an argument over who had made the right diagnosis. And who made it first.

As it turned out, the Erythromycin beat the biopsy report. After forty-eight hours on the drug, my skin lesions regressed dramatically. The negative biopsy and the positive culture for staph confirmed Dr. Steiner's *original* diagnosis of impetigo. It had been right on target.

A week later I returned to work, just as I had told Jean I would. Eva and Michael went home. My father could get back to normal, too. Which doesn't mean he stopped worrying.

* * *

In the aftermath of this episode, Dr. Steiner and Dr. Hauser undertook to reevaluate the general management of my lupus. By now, I was pleased that Syd became, by accident, my "primary" physician. How could I not appreciate that this man, who didn't know me, had dropped everything on a Saturday afternoon to see me—while Dr. Cohen, the man who was supposedly my physician, wouldn't even return my phone calls? I never saw Dr. Cohen again. There was no need to formally break my relationship with him. We'd never really had one.

My dermatological crisis yielded even more unexpected benefits. It's an old joke that "dermatologists can't kill you, but they can't cure you either." That's exactly what I needed. I didn't want someone who thought he could cure me. So Dr. Steiner not only continued to monitor my immediate—and lingering—skin problem, but also kept an eye on my lupus. He ordered more lab tests, all indicating increased disease activity. It was not possible to know whether this had been so before the impetigo, and contributing to my inability to resist the infection itself; or whether it was the result of the stress of the infection on my system, triggering a lupus flare. In any case, Dr. Steiner took the appropriate action: He increased my Prednisone for the lupus and continued to treat, if not yet cure, my skin lesions with Erythromycin.

Still, my lupus was not stable enough for me to undergo the cervical cone biopsy scheduled for late June. My system was being stressed enough by the staph infection. Dr. Klein agreed to postpone the surgery until my lupus was under better control. In the meantime, he would repeat the Pap smears to keep an eye on the dysplasia. By the end of a standard ten-day course of antibiotics my skin lesions were completely gone. Or so it seemed. I stopped taking Erythromycin and began to decrease the Prednisone. I had no trouble withdrawing from the steroids, but didn't seem to be able to do the same with the Erythromycin. A few days after stopping the antibiotic, a new lesion appeared in my armpit, just as gross and disgusting as the last batch. But this time I *knew* what it was and what to do. I called Syd, assured him that it looked *exactly* the same as the last time, and suggested that I resume taking Erythromycin—without driving up to see him.

Dr. Steiner gave me two additional instructions: Take three showers a day, with Betadine—an iodine-based antiseptic, used in hospitals as a pre-operative scrub; and go to the health center for a culture of the lesion. Although previous cultures of the lesions had shown the presence of staphylococci, Dr. Steiner wanted to be sure this was indeed the same thing. His request for a culture was more difficult to satisfy than showering with Betadine. Although I am a member of the academic staff at the university, once inside the health center I felt more like a student. All I needed was a skin culture. The receptionist was annoyed at my attempt to bypass the medical history and physical examination required for each appointment. The lab technician objected to my request to open the blister. Three nurses, two doctors, and one hour later I managed to convince someone to do that—and only that—for me. Now, I drive to Mansfield for *everything medical.* I'd rather spend the time in my car, enjoying the beauty of the scenery and the music of Vivaldi, than put up with the medical-bureaucratic idiocy of the university's health care system.

The new lesions cleared, but reoccurred each time I discontinued the Erythromycin. For the next two months it seemed as if I spent ten days on antibiotics and ten days off. It was becoming a nuisance for me, and a challenge for Dr. Steiner. Also, my inability to fully recover from the skin infection caused growing concern about my lupus. Maybe a review and reappraisal of its management was in order. My medical situation had never been so unsettled since I'd first become ill in 1968.

Thanks to Dr. Hauser, and perhaps because Syd had become as fond of me as I of him, Syd took me on as his patient. In this way I acquired a jewel of a doctor and a dear friend—while Syd soon found himself with a patient he was never going to get rid of. The result was that Syd (and Dr. Hauser, too) became so concerned about my general condition and its management that they suggested I go out of town for a consultation with a "famous" lupus specialist.

I was not keen about this idea, but saw no way out of it. The expert they referred me to was Dr. Rachel Friedman, a well-known rheumatologist noted for her research on lupus. I recognized her name from the literature I'd read. That put me one step ahead of my father. He didn't know who she was, but he didn't like the idea any more than I did. It seemed to us the venture would only be a waste of time. But so what? There was no harm in going along with the plan, if only to make Dr. Steiner and Dr. Hauser feel better. I owed them that much.

Eight

> It is common enough for people, when they fall into great disasters, to discern what is right, and what they ought to do; but there are but few who in such extremities have the strength to obey their judgment.
> —Plutarch

The summer was over. Eric had received a Fulbright award to teach in the People's Republic of China, and was about to leave the country. He would not return for a year. Accompanying him was out of the question. My precarious health would make it unwise for me to visit him. I wasn't happy about the separation, but I realized that my ill health served the useful purpose of sparing me from confronting our relationship head on. We made the typical promises lovers make when they part. Were they genuine? Or empty? A little of each? We'd had our ups and downs over the last four years, but I had always told myself Eric was "better than nothing." Now, I was about to face "nothing."

The day after Eric left, my father and I drove to Johnstown to see Dr. Friedman. The trip was more pleasant than I'd expected. My father and I hadn't been away together, alone, in several years. During my college years, while living at home, I'd grown accustomed to joining my father on some of his lecture circuits, especially to libertarian conferences. At first it bothered me to be in his "shadow," but soon I grew to feel really a part of the inner circle. The drive gave us an opportunity for some long-overdue companionship and quiet conversation. I took comfort in that. The weather cooperated wonderfully. It was a gorgeous day, cool and crisp, more like early autumn than late summer, not uncharacteristic for this part of the country. We savored the scenery, and a very good lunch, along the way.

We arrived in town late in the afternoon and checked into our hotel, a short drive from Dr. Friedman's office at the Johnstown University Health Center. I vetoed my father's suggestion to drive by the hospital on the way to the hotel, to check it out from the outside. That could wait until the morning. I had better plans for the rest of the day: a swim in the hotel's indoor pool—for my father's benefit; a shopping spree for me—the best "therapy" I know of for almost anything; and an elegant dinner out—my favorite activity, regardless of my frame of mind or health. All three turned out to be the highlights of the trip.

My appointment with Dr. Friedman was scheduled for eight o'clock the next morning. My father, even more compulsive than I, saw to it that we were at the hospital at 7:30. There was no one there. At 7:45, a receptionist appeared. There was still plenty of time to complete the paperwork that always precedes such medical exercises. Blue Cross/Blue Shield missed a great advertising slogan when American Express coined the phrase, "Don't leave home without it."

By the time I finished with the insurance forms and a lengthy questionnaire covering my medical history, the waiting room was nearly full. A few minutes after eight, the receptionist called my name. I went down a long hallway to Dr. Friedman's office. The hospital was clean and bright, more modern and elegant than Mansfield General, but not as homey as the private clinics in Asheville. There wasn't a semi-comatose body on a stretcher in sight. Nothing unpleasant so far.

I expected to be greeted by the famous Dr. Friedman herself. Instead, I was met by her "fellow," Dr. Berger. He was very young, very pleasant, and very courteous. So far so good. His initial reaction was one I had come to expect. He thought he would see a human wreck, but saw instead someone smartly dressed and vibrantly alert—someone who didn't look "sick." This, of course, is precisely the impression I *always* tried to give. As Dr. Berger probed for an understanding of the more severe manifestations of my illness, I tried my best to show him how well I had overcome the limitations imposed on me by my disease.

As I look back, it is clear I was much better prepared for this encounter than Dr. Berger. From my experience as a lupus patient, and from my desire not to be a passive recipient of the management of the disease, I could anticipate *his* moves better than he could *mine*. Sure enough, he queried me about never having had a kidney biopsy.

I knew it was coming. Amazingly, Dr. Berger insisted that a kidney biopsy be done *now*. I knew this reflected Dr. Friedman's particular interest in renal involvement in lupus. I was sure they wanted the results for their next paper, but refrained from saying so. It was enough to politely refuse the biopsy.

Once past this sticky point, I found myself in the next sandtrap: the psychiatric aspects of lupus. I was familiar with this one, too. No doctor would overlook that my parents divorced while I was a teenager and that my mother died fairly soon after. But I was not about to tell this *stranger* that I was depressed about my boyfriend's leaving the country. Dr. Berger didn't know me well enough to deserve that kind of intimate information. Nor would he have any context for interpreting it. I knew I'd never see any of the people here again.

Actually, this psychological probing aside, their interest in me, *as a person*, was nil. Zero. After several hours of conversation with Dr. Berger about my medical history, it was obvious that he was totally uninterested in how my lupus had affected my ability to get through school, or work, or *live as a human being*.

What I suspected became crystal clear. If Dr. Friedman—who barely talked to me, having delegated that job to Dr. Berger—was going to provide an evaluation of my case and a recommendation for the future management of my disease without any discussion of how I lived as a person, not just as a patient, what was the purpose of this visit? Dr. Friedman, the lupus expert, was interested only in my blood, urine, and tissue samples, not me. She had plenty of laboratory data, thanks to Dr. Steiner and Dr. Hauser, even before I arrived. She got more while I was there. In her opinion—she came in the room to offer *that*—I needed to be treated more aggressively. What she really meant was that my *lupus* needed to be treated more aggressively. Why? Because some of my laboratory tests suggested significant disease activity. How did Dr. Friedman think I should be treated? With even *higher* doses of Prednisone. But, surely, that too posed significant risks, no less serious than the disease itself.

As the day ended and the consultation with Dr. Friedman drew to its close, I was getting tired. My father, who had been silent during most of the day's activities, now spoke up.

"But Dr. Friedman, how much *more* Prednisone do you want Suzy to take?" His tone of voice bespoke incredulity and objection.

"Well . . ." Dr. Friedman paused momentarily, evidently not having thought this through. "As much as it takes to bring her complements up to normal levels."

That was it. They wanted to treat my *complement* not *me*! I was still speechless, but my father was not.

"But aren't you concerned about the side effects of the steroids? The destruction of her bones after all these years?"

I'm not sure why my father selected this from the many detrimental effects of taking steroids. As it happened, time would tell how prophetic his query was.

Again, Dr. Friedman paused, a little longer this time. She didn't expect such cross-examination—by a father-psychiatrist who fancied himself a physician no less.

"Well, doctor, that's not our major concern right now," she replied, only her form of address, but no longer her tone of voice, polite.

"Not *our* major concern" I thought? My father had the same stunned look on his face as he glanced over at me. Time to call it a day. Time for another good dinner and more shopping. We had to do something to make this "vacation" worthwhile.

At least this consultation made the medical situation in Mansfield look more encouraging. Evidently, the choice was between caring doctors and doctors who are the leaders in their field but for whom I was just another case. Unfortunately, these two desirable characteristics were, it seemed, completely incompatible. How could one find a physician equally devoted to caring for patients and committed to research? I do not belittle the value of research. Nor do I mean to suggest that a patient may not wish to submit himself to being treated by a research scientist. But if you make that choice, you may well pay the price. You may think you are serving medical science, or future generations, or some other grandiose purpose. Maybe you will be, and maybe that, in itself, serves an important purpose in *your* life. It doesn't in mine.

I could hardly wait for my next appointment with Syd, so I could relay my experiences in Johnstown to him while they were still fresh in my mind. I was not trying to boost his ego—although he may have thought so—when the first words out of my mouth were: "Syd, I'd rather have *you* for a doctor than those *experts* any day!"

* * *

About two weeks later, Dr. Friedman's report arrived as promised. Perhaps responding to my father's emphatic concern about increasing my Prednisone, Dr. Friedman offered another alternative: adding Plaquenil to my drug therapy. Actually, I had undergone a brief trial of this anti-malarial drug, often used in lupus, some ten years earlier. The theory behind adding Plaquenil is that it not only may help control the lupus, but may also allow for a reduction in the amount of Prednisone needed. The same idea of "steroid sparing" had motivated my use of Imuran. But, like Imuran, Plaquenil had its own risk/benefit ratio, its primary side effect being damage to the retinae in the eyes. Taken in a low dosage and carefully monitored by an ophthalmologist, this risk is supposedly minimal. Moreover, Plaquenil is particularly effective in controlling the skin involvement in lupus. Although I was concerned about the potential harm to my eyes, the lingering skin problem made me agree to give it a go.

There was no hurry to begin this therapy. Since it was a long-range program, waiting a little longer could do no harm. I was just about to start the busiest time at work, the beginning of the fall semester. That alone would be enough stress on my system. I didn't want to add another change to my routine. I filled Syd's prescription for Plaquenil and set it aside.

* * *

A few weeks later, I drove to Thornden for a quiet weekend. I woke up Saturday morning at my father's house and took my first dose of Plaquenil. I didn't give the extra pill a second thought. This wasn't the sort of drug that showed any benefits very quickly, nor did it produce sudden side effects.

The leaves were beginning to change colors, and I enjoyed taking in the view while horizontal on the living room couch. I spent the afternoon knitting a Christmas present for Eric. My father had been invited to a wedding reception at one of our neighbor's homes, and I decided to tag along. These particular neighbors were good friends and I'd been feeling a bit deprived in the way of any social life. I welcomed an excuse for some congenial and festive eating and drinking. I did plenty of each.

LIVING WITH IT 121

There was barely any light streaming through my bedroom window when I awoke the next morning. My whole body was shaking with the chills. It was an exceptionally warm weekend for this time of year. My father, as usual, had over air-conditioned the house during the night, one of his peculiar habits. But I knew there was more to the severe chills than could be attributed to the temperature in the room. I pulled my favorite Hungarian goose-down comforter as far up over my head as I could, leaving just enough air for me to breathe, and tried to go back to sleep. It was too early to get up anyway. I dozed off.

The next time I looked at the clock by my bed it was nearly 9:00 a.m. While asleep, I had somehow managed to throw off all the covers from the bed. My chills were gone. Instead, I now felt as if I was burning up. I got out of bed, but felt peculiarly lightheaded. I staggered into the bathroom, found a thermometer, and stuck it under my tongue. Impatient, I took it out not an instant later: 105! That couldn't be! I couldn't remember ever having a temperature that high. I decided to go back to bed, shake the thermometer down, and take my temperature again. Two minutes later, the reading was the same. I felt awful, but somehow not particularly alarmed. I decided to stay in bed for a while and wait until my father got up. Maybe by that time my temperature would be down.

My father awoke a short time later and was more than a little surprised to find me curled up in bed with a thermometer in my mouth —reading 105. When I announced that I also felt dizzy, he became alarmed. The next thing I knew, my father dashed out of the room, reappearing within seconds with a blood pressure machine in hand. As he put the tourniquet around my arm and began to take a reading I thought *he* was going to faint, judging by the look on his face. There was that red forehead, again. He took my blood pressure again, and again, and again—hoping for a more normal reading. Just like my repeated temperature taking. We were both suffering from wishful thinking. My blood pressure was frightfully low, sixty over forty, if that— suggesting I was going into shock. My father barely removed the cuff from my arm with one hand as he dialed the telephone with the other. I didn't have a chance to ask him whom he was calling, never mind stop him. Before I knew what was happening he had reached Dr. Steiner. He started blabbering in his typically nervous-father tone, even faster than in his normally rapid-fire Hungarian style.

"Syd, I'm sorry to disturb you at home on a Sunday morning, but Suzy's home and she woke up this morning with a temperature of 105. I just took her blood pressure and it's barely sixty over forty."

In minutes, I was in the car and on my way to the emergency room at Mansfield General where Syd said he would meet us. My standard argument to "wait and see" wouldn't hold this time.

Did I assume that Dr. Steiner was just humoring my father by agreeing to rush to the hospital to meet us? Perhaps. In any case, *I* didn't take the situation too seriously. Yet. As soon as we arrived, I could see that Syd was even more unnerved than my father, assuming that is ever possible. He had actually beaten us there by a couple of minutes, and rushed me through the bureaucracy as soon as I walked through the doors. After more temperature and blood pressure readings, all similar to those at home, I found myself signing an admission form with my right hand while my left was being stuck with an intravenous needle.

This was not exactly my conception of "informed consent." But, undeniably, this was a medical emergency. In view of what was staring Dr. Steiner in the face—high fever, low blood pressure, a staph infection *on top* of an underlying and somewhat unstable chronic illness—it was obvious that he had to admit me to the hospital. Still, I was *not* pleased.

By this time it was early Sunday afternoon. As an emergency room attendant wheeled me up to my room, I could overhear Syd speculating with my father about what might be wrong. His primary worry was that I had septicemia (a severe, generalized bacterial infection of the body through invasion of the bloodstream). Maybe I had experienced a reaction to the Plaquenil, however unlikely that might be. Then I overheard Dr. Steiner mention toxic shock syndrome. I did have a lingering staph infection; I was menstruating at the time; I was using tampons (although not the high-absorbancy type); and I did have a high fever and very low blood pressure. Still, that diagnosis seemed pretty far-fetched to me. If toxic shock hadn't been all over the television news and popular magazines as the "disease of the month" just then, I doubt anyone would have suggested it.

In any case, whatever the cause of the present crisis, I found myself about to undergo the obligatory forty-eight hours of "observation." So this was going to be my first experience as an inpatient. However silly it may seem, I kept thinking that I had, until now, successfully managed to evade hospitalization since my very first symptoms of lupus appeared twelve years earlier. Now my record was shattered.

When I arrived in my room, unhappy about having to be there at all, I was positively dismayed to find another person in the bed next to mine. It never occurred to me that I might be in a double room. Everything happened so fast there wasn't any time to discuss the accommodations. Even if there had been time, the outcome would have been the same. Except for a few rooms reserved for special cases *all* the patient rooms in Mansfield General are "doubles"—or larger. Why? Because it is a university hospital and when it was built, some twenty years earlier, state law mandated this interior design, allegedly as a cost-saving measure. Never mind that a *private* room at the *Mayo Clinic* costs less.

As a patient in a hospital you are stripped of autonomy and privacy just by being there. To share what small space is allotted to you with another person leaves you with no privacy whatsoever. To call such double rooms "semi-private," as most hospitals are fond of doing, is a stupid euphemism.

Perhaps I am too sensitive about needing my own space. I doubt it. Unless a family is poor, in America many children grow up having their own room, or looking forward to the time when they no longer have to share one with a sibling. While some young adults may enjoy having a roommate in college, many don't. Why else would private rooms in dormitories be regarded as rare and precious commodities? Moreover, while at college a roommate might, over time, become a good friend, this is a most unlikely benefit of a hospital double room! Yet, sick, depressed, feeling uncommunicative, you are placed in a room with a stranger. It makes no sense.

This is not my only objection to double rooms. If you are in a hospital, it is because you are sick enough to be there. You need rest. It's difficult to get any rest with all the hospital activities imposed on you. Then, when they are over, you still can't sleep when you want to—your roommate is up, watching television, chatting with visitors, or moaning in pain. Having to share a hospital room illustrates, in the most forceful way, the patient's loss of personal control in the medical world.

I was fairly lucky, however. My roommate was quiet. Her television wasn't even hooked up. She seemed to have no friends. By Sunday evening, when one of the nurses came in the room to take my vital signs, my temperature and blood pressure had returned to *normal*. I continued to receive an antibiotic drip in my IV, as a precaution. Blood cultures had been taken, but the results wouldn't be known for a day or two, at least. I closed my eyes, comfortable with the conclusion that this had all been a false alarm. I fell asleep early, tired from the day's excitement, with the unpleasant expectation that there would be a throng of doctors coming by on rounds early the next morning.

My luck in having a quiet roommate was offset by other circumstances beyond my control. No one who came in the room ever closed the door. At least once an hour a nurse came in the room, either to check on me or my roommate or to take vitals; also, a resident came during the night to draw *more* blood. It was my first night's experience with the hospital routine. I was glad I had managed to avoid it all these years.

Annoyed and restless after the third or fourth interruption and irritated by noise from the hallway, I got up to shut the door myself. Peeking out to see what all the commotion was about, I couldn't believe my eyes. An elderly janitor was heaving a large electric floor washer with big round brushes back and forth, back and forth, up and down, up and down. Surely *that* didn't have to be done at three o'clock in the morning?

By Monday morning, I was sure the worst of whatever was wrong with me was over. Syd was among the first faces to greet me. He bolted into my room around 7:00 a.m., boisterous as always, cracking jokes as usual. He didn't have an explanation for what had happened and reassured me I could leave the next day.

Unfortunately, I still had to endure a morning of hospital rounds. Mansfield General being a teaching hospital, medical students, interns, residents, and other staff physicians are there not only to take care of and treat patients, but also to learn from them. Like it or not, I was there, in part, to be studied. It's demeaning being poked and prodded and goaded into repeating "your story" to each successive group that files into the room. Nonetheless, it's better to put up with these inspections as gracefully as possible. Be polite and cooperative, and relay as much information as seems relevant. Chances are the doctors will go away satisfied and appreciative. Protesting can only backfire, and may make you a "difficult patient."

I left the hospital on Tuesday morning, forty-eight hours after checking in. I had come in with a mysterious fever and was discharged with a professional-sounding description of the same. "Diagnosis: Fever of unknown etiology." As a bonus, I took with me a mouth filled with painful, white, splotchy lesions. I'd developed a yeast infection, a typical side effect of antibiotics, especially of such massive doses as I'd received intravenously. I'd had yeast infections before, but never in *this* bodily orifice. Eating was agony. It hurt just to talk. How would I be able to answer questions all day at the reference desk in the library, or teach classes, when I could hardly speak? The answer was xylocaine, a local anesthetic, compliments of Syd. He did care about *me*, not just my disease. Xylocaine came as a gooey pink liquid. I swished it around in my mouth and it tasted awful. But it worked like a charm.

I drove straight home to Concord, anxious to be back in the library the following morning after a decent night's sleep in my own apartment. My sudden hospitalization had frightened my supervisor, Jean, and my colleagues, perhaps even more than me. Not having a telephone in my room, I hadn't been able to call anyone. Hearing the news from my father no doubt made it all sound much worse. Seeing me "looking well," as usual, once again served a useful purpose, relieving everyone's worries.

* * *

It was never determined what caused the sudden rise in my temperature and the alarming fall in my blood pressure. However, the mysterious nature of the crisis only added to Dr. Steiner's growing puzzlement over how to treat me, and my lupus, over the long run. My consultation with the "experts" in Johnstown and the emergency hospitalization escalated the uncertainty of how well controlled my lupus really was. While Syd could have stayed on permanently as my primary physician, it just wouldn't have been "right" any longer. All of us— Syd, Dr. Hauser, my father, and myself—knew this. I already had a diagnosis—lupus. For the lingering staph infection, I had Syd. I still had my coach, my father. But I had no manager. The players were restless for someone to take charge of the team. It was clear that it would be more appropriate for me to see an internist.

Actually, Dr. Hoffman was not exactly a stranger to the family.

After evading a physical examination himself for decades, my father had relented—only to appease the concern of *his* mother—and agreed to see a doctor for a belated sixtieth-birthday checkup. Who did he go to? Dr. Hoffman. Why? Because he was regarded as the best internist in town. An internist is a physician who specializes in the diagnosis and treatment of diseases of the internal organ system, making him more of a generalist than the name implies. Wasn't Dr. Hoffman exactly what we were all looking for—for *me*?

Thursday, December 4, 1980. I don't know why I remember our first date. I walked into Dr. Hoffman's office—located in a medical office building about a mile from Mansfield General—remembering, vaguely, that he was one of the physicians I'd seen on rounds during my emergency hospitalization. Indeed, I remembered him well enough to *not* place him in the large category of persons I encountered there that I never wanted to see again. Also, Syd recommended him. If Syd liked him, Dr. Hoffman must be an okay guy. My father also thought highly of him. Never one to mince words, he approved of Dr. Hoffman enthusiastically, which, considering he doesn't like many people—and is not enamored of physicians in particular—was saying a lot. My father's only significant comment, hardly meant as a criticism, was that he found Dr. Hoffman very reserved and serious, especially for someone so young. Perhaps this impression was in reaction to Syd's laid back, often flippant behavior. Maybe my father was just warning me that I shouldn't act impertinent and horse around (as I did with Syd).

Although it doesn't happen often, this time my father and I disagreed. It wasn't that I liked Dr. Hoffman any less after my first visit than he did. On the contrary. Dr. Hoffman certainly was more sober than Syd, but by no means unapproachable. Average in height, but more than average in looks, he had a quiet but cordial style. Some might say it was a little too professional. But I was accustomed to, and comfortable with, formal medical relationships. As it happened, I found Dr. Hoffman more relaxed and easy-going than I had been led to expect. I quickly realized why. My father is *much* older than Dr. Hoffman (old enough to be *his* father) and he can be pretty intimidating (at least many people think so). I am, of course, more gregarious than my father and better able to bring out the best in people, assuming there is something to bring out.

My first appointment with Dr. Hoffman focused primarily on a pre-operative physical examination. After postponing surgery for the cervical cone biopsy, the time had come to get it over with. I was as ready for it as I'd ever be. And then I did something stupid that nearly forced another delay: I cracked a rib. In fact, I didn't *do* anything out of the ordinary, which is what made the incident, however trivial, all the more troublesome. It was the day before Thanksgiving. I was sitting in the lounge in the library drinking a cup of coffee. I leaned over the side of a big wooden armchair to pick up something from the floor, and as my hand touched the floor, I heard a distinct, "CRACK." At the moment, it meant nothing to me. The next morning I realized what had happened. I spent the holiday in my apartment with a heating pad and a bottle of aspirin.

During my pre-op appointment with Dr. Hoffman, I confessed to the clumsy behavior that caused my cracked rib. The diagnosis was confirmed on X-ray. Of course, it wasn't clumsiness at all. My bones were beginning to show the ill effects of all the years of steroid therapy. They were getting thinner and more brittle. There wasn't too much I could do about it. I needed to take Prednisone. I couldn't help but recall the conversation, just a few months back, between my father and Dr. Friedman, who wanted me to take even *more* Prednisone, seemingly with no concern for just this possible, indeed probable, complication. If I had any lingering doubts about that trip being a waste of time— about recognizing that the primary interest of those researchers was to treat the disease, not the patient—now I was convinced.

My cracked rib worried the anesthesiologist more than Dr. Hoffman or me. She thought it might hamper my breathing and make her job more difficult. But the danger was not sufficient to warrant another postponement of the surgery. Besides, I'd never be the "perfect" surgical candidate.

Unlike my emergency hospitalization in September, this affair proved to be quite tolerable. I wasn't terribly worried about the operation or concerned that I might have cancer of the cervix. The fact that this time I could *plan* my hospital admission also made it less traumatic. I even managed to obtain a private room. That pleasantry would not be the only difference I'd notice between Mansfield General and the adjoining private hospital, Lyman Memorial. The latter was much older, but much cleaner. Patients were assigned *one* nurse each shift and *one* resident, instead of being checked like an automobile on an assembly

128 LIVING WITH IT

line. And the doors on the rooms stayed shut.

The surgery was uneventful. The cervical dysplasia turned out to be less impressive than my Pap smears had indicated. Because of my lupus, I received Hydrocortisone in my IV drip, to compensate for the stress of surgery. I was back at my father's house in less than a week, back in my own apartment after Christmas, and back in the library after the first of the year.

Nine

It has been a happy life. My limitations never make me sad. Perhaps there is just a touch of yearning at times. But it is vague, like a breeze among flowers. Then, the wind passes, and the flowers are content.
—Helen Keller

The next two years were, medically speaking, wonderfully uneventful. Or maybe they just seemed that way compared to the previous two. Even so, except for the onset of my illness in 1968, I had "suffered" relatively little. However progressive the *disease* might be in theory, in practice *I* was making great progress. I had completed college and obtained a graduate degree, with flying colors; I had finally moved away from home, like any other normal adult; I had a job I loved, at a prestigious university. Perhaps I treasured these achievements more than most of my friends and colleagues treasured theirs. There's no denying that the more precarious life is, the more precious it is as well.

With most of my life in order, I was anxious to establish a more secure doctor-patient relationship. For most of the past ten years—ever since Dr. Patterson, my first regular physician, left town—I had not been able to do this. Oliver Wendell Holmes once said, "What I call a good patient is one who, having found a good physician, sticks to him till he dies." I had become a pretty good patient. I needed a doctor I could "stick to." In Dr. Hoffman, I felt I had found such a physician. I knew I'd "stick to him," and he to me. Finally, I had a doctor who wasn't about to leave town for the next attractive offer that came his way.

Unlike all my previous doctors, Dr. Hoffman was in private practice. Although he had hospital "privileges" at Mansfield General and at Lyman Memorial, he was not a part of the academic medical establishment. He was likely to stay put. And his primary concern was to care for patients, not to do research on them.

From my very first visit with Dr. Hoffman I sensed both his ability and his willingness to do just that—really *care* for me, medically *and* personally. I scarcely paid much attention to it at the time, but as I now look back on the first years under Dr. Hoffman's care, I realize that I saw him more frequently than I had any doctor before him. This was the case *despite* the fact that—with the staph infection cleared and the cervical cone biopsy behind me—my lupus seemed to be under firm control. I had increased my Prednisone to 20 milligrams a day (now splitting my dosage between the morning and the evening); I stopped taking Plaquenil, reinstituted Imuran into my therapy, and hoped to cut down the Prednisone; all my laboratory tests stabilized within my own abnormal range of normal. From my perspective, it hardly seemed necessary to have an appointment every two months when there wasn't anything demonstrably wrong. After all, shouldn't one go to the doctor only when there's something awry—so he can fix it?

This approach—based on infrequent visits to the doctor simply to fix something—might be appropriate for an acute illness or injury, but it won't do in the case of a chronic illness. The chronically ill patient, however well he feels, needs to see the doctor *more* than he may like; and the physician must treat the patient, in the sense of actively doing something to him, *less* than he may like. Lest anyone think this sort of low-profile style is common among physicians, or appreciated by patients, it is not. All too often, patients want their physician to *do something*. And the physicians, eager to satisfy their clients, go along. As a result, both fail to appreciate the adage, "If it isn't broken, don't fix it."

Unfortunately, many patients and physicians find it difficult to follow this rule. Patients want to be "fixed" and doctors want to do some "fixing." The situation in medicine today is not unlike that in politics. Doing nothing is seen as a reactionary approach; whereas doing something—the activist approach—is accepted, prima facie, as "doing good." Unless the doctor (government) does something *for* you, he (government) isn't doing you any good. Nothing could be more absurd. It should come as no surprise that I am fond of the medical corollary to Thomas Jefferson's maxim that "that government is best which governs least." Indeed, centuries earlier, Hippocrates admonished physicians to "have two special objects in view with regard to disease, namely, to do good or to do no harm." The principle of laissez-faire has value in medicine no less than in politics. This, of course, does not *always* mean "letting be," leaving well enough alone. As a good conservative government must be supported by a strong, well-prepared defense force, so must all the "forces" that fight a chronic illness. Both the doctor and the patient must prepare for war if they are to enjoy peace. *Si vis pacem, para bellum.*

So far, I had been lucky, given the general disarray of my defensive medical troops. What saved me, perhaps, was that I hadn't needed to call on them. That had to change now. And that is what Dr. Hoffman and I set out to do: build a new force, slowly, together. Actually, we didn't *do* much. But that didn't lessen the value of the bimonthly appointments. We learned how to deal with one another and to trust one another. I learned to trust Dr. Hoffman enough to be able to report information to him, *as information*, without fearing he would interpret my account either as malingering, to be disdained and ignored—or as a dangerous sign of increased disease activity, to be aggressively treated. Similarly, because this honest but conservative approach was his style, he learned to trust me to be forthcoming and honestly relate relevant information when appropriate. He also learned to understand that if and when I did relate some new or unusual symptom, he'd better take it seriously, for I was able to keenly sense when there was something genuinely wrong with me. While the ability to communicate is important for any doctor-patient relationship, it was especially so for us: I lived in another city, an hour's drive away. If doctor-patient relationships are like marriages, ours exemplified the 1980s yuppie version. It was a commuter marriage.

* * *

By May of 1981—one year after the dreaded black fly bites and their aftermath—I was feeling better than I had in years. My disease as well as its overall management were under better control. Just knowing that Dr. Hoffman was standing close by made for a more tranquil situation.

It was the perfect time to celebrate, in a big way. Memorial Day 1981 was indeed memorable. But this year, unlike the last, all the memories would be wonderful. The entire family—my sister and brother-in-law, my father, his brother and sister-in-law, my grandmother and I—traveled "back to our roots" in Hungary. (Not that Michael or my uncle's wife had any roots there themselves.) Three generations, for each of whom this trip was unforgettable. My grandmother, then eighty-six years old, had nearly died (from a strangulated inguinal hernia) on her last journey to Budapest some five years earlier. My uncle had never returned since leaving the country in 1938. My sister and I had been abroad, but never to Eastern Europe. My father had been back once, a year earlier, when he was invited to give a lecture. But that trip he took with one of his girlfriends, so it didn't count for the rest of us.

Such an implausible but imaginative expedition could only have been engineered by my sister. As is her style, Eva had planned it months ahead of time, when I was still feeling quite poor. At first, I declined the offer to join the group, and agreed to go only at the very last minute. While the rest of the family, and Eva in particular, thought I was just being disagreeable, my resistance to join in the planning had a more subtle motive. After the "black fly" affair and its aftermath, I was afraid to set my hopes so high, only to have them dashed in the end. For most people, such a vacation would not seem like an unrealistic goal. For me, with the events of the previous year still fresh in my mind, with the foreboding sense that my illness was unstable, it seemed quite unrealistic. Also, I was now finally approaching a renewed feeling of medical balance; I didn't want to sacrifice it for something that seemed both frivolous and stressful. In the end, however, my desire to act like a normal person and have a good time won out over my uneasiness about suffering a relapse. Eva, too, helped immeasurably by trying to shame me into going, in her typical loving-but-browbeating older sister fashion. Last but not least, I realized that my absence would have put a damper on this pilgrimage and made it less enjoyable for everyone else. I was blessed, and I knew it, with a loving family. Everyone loved to have me around. They didn't want to go without me. I *had* to go. Besides, I'd be travelling with *three* doctors!

I hate to admit that my sister is right about anything. This time she was completely right, and I couldn't have been more wrong. It was one of her better schemes, and she carried it off masterfully.

My father, grandmother, and I flew to Boston, where we met Eva and Michael, who came in from the West Coast. Then the five of us flew to Switzerland, meeting my aunt Brigitte and uncle Andrew, who live in Zurich. From there we hopped a Malev Airlines flight to Budapest—a Hungarian plane with colorfully dressed stewardesses serving trays of greasy salami and poppyseed strudel. It was a long trip. We were all exhausted by the time we arrived at the Budapest Hilton, situated high on the hills of Buda, overlooking the Danube and the House of Parliament. Fortunately, I could regulate my jet lag with a little extra Prednisone. The next morning we were ready to roll. Sticking together required a little extra effort as no taxicab—certainly not the tiny Soviet-made Ladas—could accommodate seven persons. This meant that for each excursion, no matter how short, we needed two cars. With at least one native Hungarian speaker in each car, and lots of filterless Camels for tipping, we saw all the standard sights, along with many others of more personal interest—like my father's high school and the family's palatial ex-home. "Yinky"—Eva and I had given our grandmother this nickname when we were little, modifying "anya," the Hungarian word for mother, to our own tastes—remembered exactly where everything was, even after more than forty years.

After five days of over-sightseeing, over-drinking, and overeating, we left Budapest for Switzerland and a week in the mountains. Leaving my aunt and uncle at their home, the rest of us packed into a rented Opel and headed for Davos. Better known as a ski resort, or a summer sun-spot, it was off season at this time of year, but luckily not for the best patisserie in town. The night after we arrived, an unexpected spring snowstorm closed the mountain passes and we were happily stuck inside our hotel for a day, forced to swim in the indoor pool, play ping-pong and Scrabble, eat chocolate truffle cake, and sip champagne chilled in a pile of snow on the balcony. The next day the sun came out, the road to St. Moritz was reopened, and we witnessed, first hand, that the pictures on those Swiss calendars are *real*. All that was missing were the cows, not yet out of their stalls for the summer. Uncle Andrew loved to remind us that the cows are subsidized by the government—even in a country that is emphatically not socialist. I've never seen sky such a deep blue or mountains so majestic. Nor did I ever before have to worry about getting a sunburn in the snow! Parasol in hand, I strolled around Lake St. Moritz with Yinky and my father, while Eva and Michael raced ahead, throwing snowballs at each other and me.

How could I have seriously considered not taking this vacation? Although exhausting, the two weeks were rejuvenating. My spirits were boosted and once again I felt I could do almost anything I wanted.

*   *   *

My long-distance relationship with Dr. Hoffman continued to flourish. My long-distance relationship with Eric was another matter. When he left the country, Eric had given me power of attorney; throughout the year I kept an eye on the tenants who had sublet his apartment; we'd made plans to meet in California upon his return to the States. In September, Eric returned from China with a real surprise: a wife. I was devastated. But I was not as stunned by the news as my friends and family (or his for that matter). I had occasionally teased him that he would tire of bachelorhood and marry before he reached forty. I was right. But this was not exactly what I'd envisioned. In addition to being hurt, I felt humiliated. I've said as little as possible about Eric because I'd like to believe such relationships are no more or no less difficult to establish and maintain if one has a chronic illness than if one doesn't. I'd like to believe this, even if it isn't always true.

My having lupus was, for both of us, an easy way to evade facing our relationship more squarely. Much as I wanted to be with Eric, I would not, quite aside from my lupus, have wanted to leave my family, friends, and work. Without my illness as an excuse, I would have had to admit that Eric was not as important to me as I thought or pretended. The same, I am sure, was true for him.

In the past year we had written to each other nearly every day, and had even made a few expensive trans-Pacific telephone calls. My reaction to his marriage announcement, I suppose, was quite ordinary: anger, hurt, disappointment, rejection. I found myself losing sleep and overworking. Before long, I felt fatigued, achy, and ill. A year earlier I had used my lupus as a legitimate excuse for not accompanying Eric to China; now I used it as an illegitimate excuse for feeling lousy. After all, weren't these the classic symptoms of increased disease activity? If they signalled lupus, I would not be responsible for them. But if instead they were the symptoms of lovesickness, I, and only I, would be responsible for them. I'd never considered playing the sick-therefore-not-responsible role before.

Fortunately, I quickly snapped out of this mental state and admitted to myself that "it" was lovesickness, not lupus-sickness. I also knew that my self-imposed stress could precipitate a *real* exacerbation of the disease. In order to avoid a true relapse, I needed to come to grips with my feelings of depression and fatigue, feelings I was entitled to as much as any healthy person.

With the fall semester well under way, it was easy enough to busy myself in my work, which I loved. But I felt I needed something else to help me get over Eric. Being with my friends or my family, supportive though they were, was also not enough. Indeed, their ever-ready support was marred by the fact that they kept telling me that Eric was exploiting me, that he was not giving me enough, that I was doing too much for him. Some just said he was a jerk and that I was much better off without him. Even if all this was true, such comments did not help my own sense of worth. I still took attacks on Eric's character as attacks on my own judgment.

I needed to meet some new people, do something new for a change. I decided to get involved in politics again. I had worked as a volunteer on local and national election campaigns, on and off, ever since the presidential race of 1968, when I was only thirteen. Many of my eighth-grade classmates were already initiated into the political world, thanks to close relatives who were candidates, and at that time my political leanings meshed with those of my peers. While my main motive then was to go along with my friends' activities, my main motive now was to get away from my friends. This was easy enough. In my present circle of acquaintances in Concord, I didn't know a soul who shared my libertarian-Republican political philosophy. When I decided to lend my help to the Republican candidate in the mayoral race, the kindest reaction I received—from those to whom I dared tell what I was doing—was ridicule. I was wasting my time. To everyone's surprise, "my" candidate beat the Democratic incumbent—in a town that was, and still is, a liberal holdout from the 1960s.

Perhaps naively, I assumed that my friends would accept my political persona as a part of who and what I am, just as they accepted my medical persona. I considered both my illness and my politics as personal matters (if I were religious, I would add my faith to the list), shared only with close friends. Since I hadn't experienced ostracism because of my illness, I didn't expect to be shunned because of my political beliefs. I was wrong. I came to understand that people feel compelled to have sympathy for those in ill health, because the sick are not responsible for their condition—but are under no such compulsion when they confront those whose political (or religious) persuasions differ from theirs, precisely because the latter are indeed responsible for their beliefs. I have no objection to genuine sympathy or to sincere intellectual disagreement. But I find both offensive when the person offering sympathetic words does it only to make himself feel better, and the person engaging in intellectual debate does it only to make himself feel superior.

"Accepting" persons with chronic disabilities is now one of the favorite pastimes of otherwise frequently narrow-minded Americans. Proffered on the premise of tolerance, attempts to "mainstream" the handicapped are largely self-satisfying. Television "telethons" focused on raising money for a particular disease or disability exhibit a hideously patronizing approach. They emphasize how different the diseased and disabled are from normal, healthy people—typically, by displaying the victims on the screen. The fact that these campaigns are waged most enthusiastically for diseases and disabilities which can be *visibly* portrayed illustrates how much the "normals" want to *see* themselves as better off than the "abnormals."

When the elections were over, I began to think more about my work at the library. Although I enjoyed my work as a reference librarian in the undergraduate library of a large university, I felt I needed a change of pace. My job required long hours, the intensity of the work fluctuating with the college calendar. I was not one of those librarians who sits behind her desk all day, if there are any such. I wasn't bored. But the job was becoming more of a physical than an intellectual challenge.

I needed something to perk me up. Any other twenty-six-year-old woman dropped by a boyfriend would have set her sights on landing a new beau. I figured I was better off going after something with greater promise of success. I was always more confident about my brains than my looks. This time I was smart enough to see opportunities that stared me in the face: a position as reference librarian in the graduate research library. The job seemed to offer the best of all possible worlds—a chance for new and more challenging work, without having to move from Concord. I didn't want the stress of relocating, making new friends—finding another doctor!

I applied, interviewed, and waited—along with other candidates from around the country. I got the job. In February 1982 I started work in my new position. As the new year got under way, I felt much better about myself—physically, personally, and professionally—than I had at the end of 1981. I did begin to wonder if I'd ever have another date.

But I took solace in seeing many of my single *healthy* female colleagues in a similar situation. As for those who were not unattached, I concluded I was better off than most, judging from the company they kept.

In April 1982, I learned that my last regular gynecological examination had revealed a cervical polyp (a growth that can protrude from any membranous surface). I would need to undergo a "D&C." This is so common a procedure that even its abbreviated name is generally understood, although perhaps not everyone knows it stands for dilation (stretching out) of the cervix and curettage (scraping) of the lining of the uterus. The process is both therapeutic, in that it removes the undesired growth or tissue (in this case a polyp), and diagnostic, in that the removed tissue can be examined microscopically for possible malignancy. Naturally, I wondered if this procedure could wait until the end of the semester when my absence from work would be less of a strain on my colleagues—and less of a blot on my record. I was relieved when I was told I could wait. I was more relieved when I was told I wouldn't have to spend even one night in the hospital! The D&C could be performed in what was then a relatively new facility—an outpatient surgery center.

Outpatient surgery has become popular since then, mainly for economic reasons. It frees up hospital beds for those in more serious need; it saves the patient time and aggravation; and, most of all, it saves the insurance companies money. D&C's, dental extractions, minor eye surgery, tonsillectomies, abortions, and tissue biopsies are among the most common procedures performed in outpatient surgery settings. The practice allows the patient to come to the surgery center early in the morning, undergo the procedure, rest for several hours under observation, and return home by early afternoon or the end of the day.

It sounded good to me. I didn't like being hospitalized. The prospect of being able to return home (to my father's house at least) the day of surgery—to sleep in my own bed in my own room—sounded too good to be true. I wondered how my health insurance would cover this. I didn't have much doubt that it would be covered by my Blue Cross/Blue Shield policy. The policy had so far paid for all my outpatient laboratory work and my two hospitalizations. Still, unacquainted as I was with outpatient surgery, I decided I'd better re-read the policy, instead of taking for granted that it covered everything.

I didn't discover anything unexpected. Not in my Blue Cross file.

But next to it, I noticed another folder marked "Medical Insurance—Miscellaneous." There sat my in-hospital cash plan policy. Although I had been paying the premiums faithfully since my father had talked me into purchasing the policy more than five years earlier, I had completely forgotten about it! I didn't even remember exactly what it was for. Would it serve any purpose now? Since the surgery center, by definition, was not "in-hospital," the answer was no. The basic requirement for a claim was spending at least one night *in* the hospital. But wait a minute. Was this *all* that was required? I read on. Indeed it was. So why hadn't I claimed any benefits for my two hospitalizations in September and December of 1980? Because I had forgotten that I *had* such a policy! And so had my father! And now it was *too late* to file a claim.

Now that I remembered, I almost wished the D&C was scheduled to be performed *in* the hospital. Almost, but not quite. The comforts of my father's house far outweighed any cash benefits paid for enduring less pleasant accommodations. Despite newspaper and television stories citing abuses of in-hospital insurance policies by would-be patients, I cannot imagine many people subjecting themselves to needless nights in a hospital in order to make money, nor many physicians collaborating in such schemes.

Mandatory outpatient surgery for certain procedures—that is, mandatory if you want your insurance company to pay the bill, as was the case for my D&C—does have one negative consequence. Underlying the idea of outpatient surgery is the assumption that you are well enough not to require hospitalization and can recuperate at home. But what if you live alone? I did. Fortunately, I was able to go to my father's house. Many single adults don't have such an option. Without family or a close friend to take care of you, you are faced with a difficult, and potentially costly, dilemma. In some ways, then, outpatient surgery, like certain sophisticated medical therapies, focuses only on the disease to be treated—not the personal circumstances of the individual patient.

My outpatient surgery was uneventful, an insignificant addition to my repertoire of medical experiences. The results of the biopsy still showed some dysplasia, as expected from the Pap smears. But Dr. Klein was confident that he had removed the affected tissue. And with the Imuran discontinued, he felt that the chance of these abnormal cells being cancerous was minimal.

LIVING WITH IT 139

I returned to the library after a long weekend at home, glad the spring semester was over. I looked forward to a real vacation with my father later in the summer. We planned to fly to San Francisco, spend a week driving down to Carmel and Monterey, then back up through the Napa Valley vineyards and on to Bodega Bay, and return to San Francisco via the northern coast. I was also eager to start my new assignment at work come fall. I would be responsible for hiring, training, and supervising the dozen student assistants in the Reference Department.

I always liked having occasions and goals ahead of me. And I was content to have my life in order again.

Ten

"Thank you, whatever comes." And then she turned
And, as the ray of sun on hanging flowers
Fades when the wind hath lifted them aside,
Went swiftly from me. Nay, whatever comes
One hour was sunlit and the most high gods
May not make boast of any better thing
Than to have watched that hour as it passed.
—Ezra Pound

January 1983 was a typical January in Concord. It was slow in the library, with most of the students away for intersession—a time to catch up with unfinished work and get some rest. But this New Year didn't start off as restfully as I'd hoped it would. I didn't realize how hectic the holidays had been until I returned to my apartment in Concord feeling more in need of a vacation than when I had arrived in Thornden Christmas Eve.

I'm sure I would have spent my first weekend alone curled up on the sofa with a good book if the normally dismal weather in Concord had cooperated. But, unexpectedly, it was June in January. The temptation to throw off the heavy coats and boots, put on a light sweater, and go hiking in one of the local state parks was too much to resist. The trail through the gorge to the waterfall was a mile long. I was nearly at the end when I realized there was no short way back to the beginning. There was no choice but to keep walking. It would be my last hike for more than a year. Of course, I didn't know that then.

* * *

I awoke the following Saturday morning feeling unusually achy. I took two aspirin and a long, hot shower. I spent the day in my apartment. Next to the top floor of a highrise building, it offered a spectacular view of the campus and the hillside surrounding Concord. Like living in a lifesize landscape painting, today it was a snowscape by Monet or Pissaro. After twenty-four hours of rest, and another half-dozen aspirin, I felt worse. I was achier and feverish. My temperature was 101. I went back to bed.

Monday morning, January 24, I should have been in the library, teaching my first class of the semester. With my temperature now at 102, I called in sick, announcing in the same breath that I'd be in the next day. I didn't want to drive fifty miles through the snow to see Dr. Hoffman. Instead, I called his office to inform him of my symptoms.

"This is Suzy, may I speak to Jill, please?" I didn't need a last name to get past the receptionist to Dr. Hoffman's nurse. "I'm just calling to tell you I'm sick and plan to stay home from work today. Temperature 102. Sniffles. Everyone seems to have it. . . . NO, I don't need to talk to *him*. I think I'm better off resting than driving up to see him. Right?"

"I'll talk to Dr. Hoffman and see what he says. Be sure to call me back if you get any worse. And call back by the end of the week anyway, just to let us know you're better."

It was our usual routine. I felt comfortable calling in, knowing I wouldn't be asked to come in for a perfunctory examination, yet knowing I could see Dr. Hoffman immediately if I needed to.

Unable to fall back asleep, I moved to the sofa, and tried to figure out what was going on. A temperature of 102, while not especially alarming in a normal person, is unusual in someone taking steroids. And while I regularly ran a low-grade fever (a common symptom in lupus), it rarely rose this high. Indeed, the last time I'd had a significant fever was in the fall of 1980, when I was hospitalized for my supposed case of toxic shock. On the other hand, many people at work were sick, with flu-like illnesses and high fevers. Perhaps that was all I had, too. I didn't feel terribly ill. I was achy and tired, but had no sore throat, and only a slight cough and the sniffles.

The next thing I knew, I awoke from a deep sleep. It was pitch dark outside. The sun sets early in January, but I could hardly believe I had slept away the whole day. I must have needed the rest. Still, it made me anxious that I had done this. Perhaps it was a sign of something serious. I got up, washed my face, and made some scrambled eggs and an English muffin—my favorite "sick food"—and returned to the sofa to watch the evening news on television.

I had promised to be back at work the next day. Foolishly, I kept my word. As I readied myself for the day, I felt light-headed, but attributed it to too much sleep, too much television, and not enough food. It was nothing a good day's work wouldn't cure. A bottle of aspirin and an extra sweater in my bag, I was in the library at 8:00 a.m.

* * *

Whether it was the frenzy at work that first week of the spring semester, or the high level of aspirin in my system, or both—the work week just disappeared. I had planned to drive to Mansfield for the weekend, to attend the wedding of a high school classmate. My father was out of town, as he frequently was, so I decided to treat my grandmother to an elegant dinner out Friday evening, and then stay at her house that night.

Actually, I didn't like staying at Yinky's house, and did so only rarely. This time, it made good sense. I'd be alone at my father's house in Thornden, farther from the church where the wedding was to take place, and the weather was lousy. It was simply a matter of convenience, although I tried to make it look more like love for my grandmother. I'm sure she could see through all this. She knew how I felt about staying at her house. It brought back memories of staying there, with Eva, many years earlier, when our parents were about to divorce. Not the best of times. Not the best of memories. It had nothing to do with Yinky, then or now. She was an innocent bystander. But, try as she might, the memories of that time, that house, have never faded. When I looked at the situation objectively, and could see how hurt Yinky was by this lingering mental association, I would try to forget the past and stay with her. I knew how much this gesture, however infrequent, meant to her. Sadly, for both of us, this weekend would be the beginning of a new set of even more traumatic memories connected with her house.

The next morning the alarm rang at 9:00, an uncivilized hour for a Saturday. It was time to get up and get ready for the wedding. I felt as if I had barely enough strength to shut off the clock. My head was throbbing, my nightgown was sopping wet, and I was shivering. When I threw off the covers from the bed I noticed that the sheets and pillows were soaked. At my father's house, I was subjected to his overcooling the place at night. At Yinky's, it was the opposite. But I knew I couldn't blame the way I felt on the thermostat, even if it was set at seventy-four. Yinky looked at me as if I were a ghost. Instead of saying "Good morning," I greeted her with, "Do you have a thermometer?" I knew without taking it that I had a high fever. Yinky returned with the thermometer and I stuck it under my tongue while I watched my tea get darker. Tea instead of coffee—for me, another symptom of feeling poorly. Chilled and clammy, I was in a hurry to take a sip, and removed the thermometer after only a few seconds.

"How much is it?" Yinky asked, anxiously. It wasn't the last time I would be angered by her inquisitiveness—understandable, but annoying nevertheless. Or by her grammar. Yinky's English is nearly perfect by any standard, especially considering that she learned the language when she was middle-aged. But she had picked up certain expressions which, though not incorrect or unconventional, sounded "uneducated," lower class. It did no good to point these out. My father and I had tried. It only made her use them more frequently.

I was too tired to argue or lie, so I blurted out, "Almost 103. I guess I'm not going anywhere today."

"Aren't you going to call the doctor?" she demanded.

I yelled back, "NO," without feeling the need to justify my answer. Actually, I didn't need to be concerned about disturbing Dr. Hoffman at home. About six months before he had given up his solo private practice and joined a group of five other internists. This arrangement provided for one of the six physicians to be on call twenty-four hours a day. It was reassuring to know I could always reach someone from the office, with a 16.7 percent chance of reaching Dr. Hoffman himself. But I'd never called "the service" before. I saw no reason to, yet.

Although I had no intention of leaving the house, I took a shower, washed my hair, put on makeup, and changed into one of Yinky's clean nightgowns. Getting dressed in real clothes seemed pointless. But the rest of the ritual was not without purpose. The shower, the hair, the makeup—these activities were necessary for my own sense of well-being. And for appearances. I wanted to distance myself from how lousy I felt. I also wanted to reduce my grandmother's anxiety. I didn't need to apply blush to my cheeks. They were rosy enough.

This exercise in self-improvement took much longer than it normally does. I was slowed down not only by the slightly unfamiliar surroundings but by the repeated need to stop and rest. When I completed the task and entered the living room, I knew the effort was successful. *I* didn't feel better, but I managed to make Yinky feel better. I could tell by the look on her face that she was convinced I wasn't so sick after all.

My makeup and hair were of no help, however, when my father called that evening. The sound of my voice was enough for him. Also, with my father I never hid my true feelings. We had grown as close as we had largely because we were so open and honest—and critical— of one another. Hardly a paper from high school or college hadn't passed before his judgmental eye and revisionist pencil before coming back with an "A." Likewise, he rarely sent off a letter to the editor, much less an article or a book, without my attacking it with a red pen. Forthright opinions were equally frank and frequent concerning non-academic affairs, especially of the heart. In a way, I became the stereotypical daughter of a single father, he the protective father of the youngest daughter. Well, maybe not so typical. We went further than father and daughter in our candor about our feelings. When it came to my health, I always put all my cards on the table for him, and he with me. That didn't mean I always listened to what he had to say. Well, I did always *listen*. I just didn't always act accordingly. Many an "I told you so" followed. But so did an occasional "I guess I was wrong—that *wasn't* too much for you after all."

Tonight's conversation, then, was not so uncommon. I gave him a report, both medical and personal. "Temperature 103. I feel like shit. No, I can't be more specific." A minor debate followed over the pros and cons of calling Dr. Hoffman's service before the weekend was over, but my father eventually agreed that I was better off resting until Monday morning. I could call Dr. Hoffman at the office then.

I spent the remainder of the weekend doing just that—resting. It was difficult to keep changing from wet night clothes without Yinky noticing, but I managed by alternating the two gowns I had. In the overheated house, they dried out quickly. With my father on my side, I no longer had to argue with my grandmother about calling The Doctor. But this time my father and I had not been entirely candid with each other. We both sensed, right then, that something was seriously wrong with me. Of course, neither of us had any idea what.

* * *

I called the library on Monday morning, as I had the week before. I was now starting to lose my voice, having developed a dry, unproductive cough. It was a struggle to say, "Hi, Kelly? Is Judith in yet?" I deliberately telephoned early, knowing my supervisor would be late. It was easier to tell the secretary I wasn't coming to work, although the sound of my "hello" conveyed a good deal more.

"You sound *awful*! Where *are* you?"

"Still at 'home.' I'm feeling worse. My temperature is up to 103. I'm going to call the doctor and try to see him today. I doubt I'll be back this week." The words rang in my ears: "This week." A week before I had called in and convincingly claimed I'd be out only a day. I knew better this time. "Kelly? I guess I'd better talk to Elizabeth about the desk schedule, and Linda about the classes I'm supposed to teach this week." I was more concerned about work than my health as I waited for one or both of them to get on the line.

Elizabeth sounded more worried about me than the schedule, despite her abrupt, "No problem, I'll take you off all week, and if you make it back sooner, we'll put you back on."

Linda was clearly terrified at the thought of teaching two of my classes.

"Are you okay?" she inquired, politely. "Can you tell me where you left your notes?"

I felt like laughing, but didn't.

"Do you mean you don't have any?" she continued, after a long pause.

I did the best I could, my voice notwithstanding, to talk her through an outline. Fortunately, Kelly interrupted our conversation to tell me she'd take care of the student assistants' schedules, the worst of my duties. I'd talked long enough. I wanted to lie down.

"I'll call you in a couple of days and let you know what's happening. Thanks, guys."

I could tell there was more than one person on the other end of the line. My head was spinning. Just talking about work seemed to add to my fatigue.

Jill wouldn't be in at Dr. Hoffman's office until nine. I might as well have breakfast and make myself presentable before calling. That way I'd be ready to go. I knew I'd have to.

* * *

"Can you come in NOW? I can squeeze you in before his first patient." I don't think Jill even looked at Dr. Hoffman's schedule. A temperature of 103 plus the sound of my voice was all she needed to hear. "I thought you were better since you didn't call back last week!"

"I tried to talk myself out of it, but it didn't work. Yes, I can be there shortly. The roads don't look great, but I'm at my grandmother's house, so it shouldn't take me more than fifteen minutes."

As soon as I got off the phone, I felt as though all I wanted to do was lie down again and go back to sleep. Driving the few miles to Dr. Hoffman's office seemed an insurmountable task. Not wanting to let my guard slip in front of Yinky, I stared out the big picture window in her living room at the cars sliding about and suggested she call a cab. I knew that, to her, not wanting to drive in this weather would be a sign of good sense rather than of ill health.

Like my father, Dr. Hoffman was not one to be easily fooled by a little makeup. He looked over my chart as we talked, mulling over the notes detailing my call of a week ago. He did a complete physical, listened to me breathe, poked around, took a chest X-ray—and acted more pensive than usual. There was little else for him to do, other than send me to the lab for blood work and urinalysis. His puzzled look intensified as my cough became incessant. He glanced again at my chart.

"It's really been more than a week now that you haven't been feeling well, right?"

I stopped to think a minute before answering. "I guess if I count from the very beginning, it *has* been that long. To tell you the truth, I've never felt this awful, this drained. I wish I could describe it better."

Dr. Hoffman paused for a moment, although I don't think there was much doubt in his mind what he would prescribe next.

"I think you should increase your Prednisone to 25 milligrams; 15 in the morning and 10 in the evening. This has been enough stress on your system already, and I suspect there may be some smoldering lupus activity underlying this respiratory infection. We'll have to see the results from the lab to be sure, but let's go ahead with this now. You're staying in town for a while, I assume?"

His last words sounded more like an order than a question. I nodded in agreement, as if to say, "I'm not *that* crazy," and got up from the examining table, steadying myself so as not to look as dizzy as I felt.

Dr. Hoffman gave me his usual pat on the back with one hand, and a slip for the lab with the other. "If you want to take something for the fever, take Tylenol instead of aspirin. And let me know if it goes any higher."

Again, I nodded in agreement. I was too tired to ask what difference it made if I took Tylenol or aspirin.

"Call me back later this week—sooner if you feel worse."

* * *

My father returned from his trip on the lecture circuit late Thursday, in time for a sumptuous Hungarian feast at Yinky's. He seemed surprised and relieved that I "didn't look that sick." But when I turned away my portion of one of Yinky's best desserts, "palacsinkas"—crepes filled with apricot jam, smothered with warm, bittersweet chocolate sauce— he knew there was something seriously wrong with me. I followed this unprecedented action with another: I announced that I was too tired to drive to his house, and wanted to spare myself the long drive back into town to Dr. Hoffman's office in the morning. "I'd rather stay here," I mumbled, exhausted and half asleep.

Before my father left for home, we reviewed the medical report, such as it was, one more time. The lab results had now come back and showed evidence of a slight increase in lupus activity, but nothing alarming. The chest X-ray was normal. The urinalysis was normal. Perhaps it was just the flu. But, never one to stay out of the medical action, my father suggested a new treatment. "Why don't you ask 'Hoff' about taking some Erythromycin for the respiratory infection?"

Ever since my slow, but successful, cure of the staph infection, Erythromycin had become more than just the antibiotic of choice in our house. It was now part holy water, part placebo.

Despite nearly a week's rest, I was still tired when I called Jill

Friday morning. How I had hoped each morning that I would wake up feeling just a little bit better than the day before. Instead, each morning I felt worse. And the worse I felt, the less able I was to describe exactly what I meant. The only thing that had changed since Monday was that now, on top of the utter exhaustion, I had no appetite. Perhaps not a peculiar symptom for others, it was certainly unusual for me.

"Jill? No, I'm not any better. I'm DEAD tired. Maybe from too much sleep!" It was hard to joke about this, but I tried.

"With the weekend coming, I think Dr. Hoffman will want to see you again," Jill responded. "Is two o'clock okay?"

This appointment was a repeat of Monday's. I recounted my symptoms. Dr. Hoffman did a physical examination, ordered a chest X-ray, and sent me to the lab. It seemed to me he was tired, too, and perplexed about how to proceed. It was the perfect moment to interject my father's opinion. I think Dr. Hoffman agreed to the Erythromycin for lack of any better ideas. He wrote a prescription for 250 milligrams, four times a day—the standard dosage. He also increased my Prednisone to 30 milligrams a day.

"If you aren't any better soon, we're going to have to think about admitting you to the hospital," he announced as our meeting came to a close. "And ask Jill to give you an appointment for Monday."

I could tell Dr. Hoffman was not in the mood for banter. And I saw something else I'd never seen before: There was no sparkle behind his otherwise stern glance, even for me. There was only worry. I knew this was getting serious. I sensed he had already decided to admit me to the hospital. There just wasn't much point in pushing me to go in on a Friday afternoon.

I bundled myself up for the bone-chilling cold and climbed into a cab. In less than half an hour I was back in bed at Yinky's. I vowed to stay put for the weekend—as if I had the energy for anything else. My determination to get good rest was also driven by an intense desire to avoid going to the hospital. More sleep, forty-eight hours of Erythromycin, and my father around for the next few days. Surely I would be better by Monday.

I wasn't. Again, I awoke drenched in sweat, shaking with the chills, and my head pounding. My temperature was now inching past 103. And the increased steroid dosage had not even given me its customary agitated "hyper" effect I sometimes found annoying, but would have welcomed now. On the other hand, I did experience the expected side effect of the Erythromycin—nausea. I dragged myself into the bathroom and stood in the shower, the water running as long and as hot as I could bear it.

I was quite surprised when Dr. Hoffman didn't insist I be admitted to the hospital that very afternoon. Instead, he agreed to one more reprieve. He suggested doubling the antibiotics to 500 milligrams, four times a day, and said I could stay at home so long as my temperature didn't hit 104. It was the best deal I could have hoped for.

* * *

"Hello, this is Miss Szasz. I'm one of Dr. Hoffman's patients and I've been sick for a couple of weeks now. He told me to call in if my temperature reached 104, and it's now about 105. I can wait until the morning."

My father had left town for another lecture, contracted long before, that he didn't want to cancel on short notice. I was still at Yinky's. I was sicker than ever. Obviously, I *had* to go the hospital. To make matters worse, it was eleven o'clock at night. I had to call the *service*. What a time to see how it worked!

"We'll check with the doctor on call and have him get right back to you. What's your number there?"

It couldn't have been more than a minute before the phone rang.

"Dr. O'Donnell here. Susan? I think you'd better come right in. I'll meet you in the emergency room."

There was no way out of this now. Before I could say, "I'll have to call a cab," he went on to say that an ambulance was on its way. AMBULANCE?

The ambulance arrived so quickly I barely had time to tell Yinky what was happening. Unfortunately, I couldn't convince her to stay at home. When the crew—a young woman about my age and size and a slightly older man nearly six feet tall and three hundred pounds—came to the door, they seemed confused to find me, the patient, looking un-sick, arguing with this fragile, worried-looking *very* old woman. For a second, I was sure they wondered which of us was the patient! Much to my disappointment, they said it would be fine for my grandmother to come along. I insisted I didn't need to be carried out on a stretcher.

I could walk just fine. As a matter of fact, I was more concerned about my grandmother's slipping on the icy driveway, breaking a hip and landing in the hospital herself. I went on my own steam, accompanied by the young woman. I left the big guy to hold onto Yinky.

We were in the emergency room at Lyman Memorial in minutes. Dr. O'Donnell was waiting for me. I was wheeled into an examining cubicle with a retinue of medical personnel and equipment in tow. Then, with an IV in my left arm, I was sent off to what can only be described as a staging area to wait for an empty hospital bed.

By one a.m. I was prepared for a long, uncomfortable night on a stretcher. I finally managed to convince Yinky there was no point in *both* of us spending a sleepless night in this holding tank.

A night in a hospital emergency room is an experience no one needs. It's not that it's boring. I got plenty of attention myself, and then there was the drama of the other patients. On the far side of the room lay a woman who, it seemed, was there because an "acquaintance" of hers had beaten her up. This hypothesis was confirmed when the assailant stormed in to try and "talk some sense" into her. I was glad I was at the opposite end of the room. Between her and me, and two sets of curtains, lay a delirious man. He rambled incessantly but I couldn't figure out what he was saying. While curtains create a semblance of physical privacy, they don't conceal conversation. So when the resident on call came to examine him, I overheard that he had attempted suicide, by swallowing a bottle of dry gas. In Florida, he might have had more joie de vivre, perhaps. On my other side lay an old man, moaning, his wife at his side. He'd had a stroke. All this time I was wide awake and very uncomfortable, lying on a hard stretcher without even a pillow under my head. My temperature had soared to 105.9.

Despite all the commotion, I must have eventually dozed off. It was early morning and Dr. Hoffman was standing by my "bed."

"The first thing we have to do is find you a room. They're all filled right now. But there will be some discharges this morning. Hopefully by noon. I'll come back to see you when you're upstairs."

It was past noon by the time I settled into Room 6036, after twelve hours in the emergency room. I didn't care that I had missed lunch, especially when I discovered that I was in a PRIVATE room. It was a nice room, on one of the corners of Lyman Memorial, overlooking the campus of Mansfield University and much of the downtown of the city. It was probably one of the best rooms in the hospital. It was close to the nurses' station and kitchen, where I soon learned I could always find toast, hot tea, soda, juice—and ice. The ice became especially important as my temperatures continued to peak at 105 and I used the ice, in various ways, to cool down. I had my own bathroom, my own shower, a small closet, a chair for visitors, the standard wall-mounted television, and a telephone.

I had waited days to call the library, hoping to have better news. Instead, I now had to report that I was in the hospital and had no idea when I would be back at work.

Then it struck me that I had forgotten about Yinky! She was probably beside herself by now, not having heard anything since I'd sent her home from the emergency room in the middle of the night. I knew she'd come to the hospital as soon as I called. Maybe that's why I had "forgotten." I really didn't want her here. It wouldn't do me any good to have her sitting by my bedside, holding vigil, looking nervous. Still, it wasn't fair of me not to call.

I tried to sound cheerful, even though I didn't feel that way. "Surprise! I finally got into a room, just now." I was lying by only a few hours. "I missed out on lunch by the time I got settled into my room—6036. Why don't you bring me some 'paderevsky'?"

I wasn't really hungry, but the sight of these cookies—another of Yinky's Hungarian specialties, a wicked mixture of butter, ground walnuts, and raspberry jam, on which Eva and I had bestowed this private name—might help my spirits if not my appetite. I could always count on Dr. Hoffman, who had a sweet tooth to match mine, to help me eat them. And just asking for the cookies made Yinky feel better.

By the time Dr. Hoffman reappeared in the afternoon, he had already seen several reports from the lab. Most of the test results sounded familiar and not especially abnormal, for me. They rekindled my hope that fever or no fever, perhaps this hospitalization wasn't necessary. But I was wrong. "Your platelet count is 109,000," Dr. Hoffman concluded.

This was the last test Dr. Hoffman mentioned and it was one I understood without further explanation. Platelets, produced in the bone marrow, are essential to the blood clotting process. The fewer one has, the more prone one is to bruise and bleed. I had always bruised easily and hadn't noticed anything unusual lately. But I knew that this figure was significantly below the normal range of 150,000 to 300,000.

"That doesn't sound so good, does it? So, *now* what?"

Somewhere during the long pause that followed, my father appeared in the room. What timing. He had just returned from his latest trip and learned of my whereabouts when he called his mother. Dr. Hoffman could fill him in on the numbers shortly. I didn't need to hear them again so soon. I wanted to be filled in on the plan of action. Dr. Hoffman laid out phase one, now appearing a bit intimidated by my father's presence.

"We need to rule out any underlying infection. We'll take some blood cultures and leave the antibiotic drip in the IV for at least another day."

"What type of antibiotics?" my father chimed in, as if to remind Dr. Hoffman that this had been his idea in the first place, when he suggested I take Erythromycin. I wondered, what is this, a test?

"Cephalosporin, Kefzol, and Gentamicin," Dr. Hoffman responded. That kept my father quiet for the moment. "We'll raise the Prednisone from 30 to 45 milligrams a day. I also think we should stop the Imuran. And we'll run some tests to rule out infection."

It was clear that I was going to be here for some time. Neither my father nor I dared ask just how long. Dr. Hoffman didn't volunteer an opinion. I doubt he had one.

"I'll see you in the morning," he said as he left the room. I could never have imagined how often I'd hear that line, or how much his visits would come to mean to me.

My father and I were finally alone, but by now I was too exhausted to make good use of our time together. There was one thing, however, that couldn't wait any longer. I was glad he was there to call Eva and Michael with the news. They knew I hadn't been well the last few weeks, but we hadn't spoken any more frequently than usual. I wasn't in the mood to argue with them over the merits of my being hospitalized, much less the plan of treatment, such as it was. They always managed to find fault with the doctors in Mansfield and with the way my illness was being treated. They spoke to my father while I dozed off.

* * *

My initiation into the morning routine of the hospital began on Friday morning. A lab technician awakened me to draw blood; next, a scale was dragged in to weigh me; finally, my vital signs were checked. Of course, no nurse would ever tell you what your blood pressure, pulse, or temperature was. But after filling in the chart, the nurse would hang it on the bulletin board on the wall across from the bed. It was easier to get up and read it after she left the room than ask her to compromise her "professionalism." My own morning ritual followed: shower, hair, makeup. Patients don't get "dressed" in the hospital, so these preliminaries were the closest I could come to imitating my daily routine at home. Usually, I could complete my toilette before the main attraction of the morning: rounds.

My first day was big on rounds. I felt as though I was the most interesting case to check into Six North in weeks. This was true. More important, not only was I a diagnostic mystery, I could also talk. I mean not just literally, not being comatose, but in the sense that I could converse fairly well in medicalese. This endeared me to many of the senior physicians who would come by, and put the medical students in a state of awe, as I often knew more than they did. However, this same characteristic often did me more harm than good when it came to dealing with the vast number of doctors in the middle of the hierarchy: interns and residents. No doubt they saw me as a threat, a patient meddling in their business, and they were more interested in impressing their own superiors, and themselves, than in listening to me.

After forty-eight hours, a half-dozen temperature spikes of 105, and futile attempts to bring it down with cold washcloths (which did more to soak the bed than cool me down), I was subjected to a more sophisticated chilling procedure—a "hypothermia blanket." Two nurses stripped the blanket and sheets from my bed and replaced them with a thick, black, rubber "mattress." It looked like a rubber raft. They filled it with a mixture of cold water and ice cubes. Then I had to lie down on it. It was agonizingly uncomfortable. Because of the huge surface area compared to the washcloths, the "blanket" did cool me down a lot more quickly. Fortunately, I wasn't tied down to the bed and could get up occasionally. Nevertheless, I decided my first experience with this dreadful contraption would also be my last. It was absurdly unpleasant. There had to be a better way to cool down. I figured out a way to make relatively leak-proof ice bags by filling standard hospital rubber gloves with ice from the kitchen and tying the wrists into knots, making a balloon. It worked. The nurses went along. I prepared the balloons, and they didn't have to change the sheets three times a day.

The first weekend also produced my first visitors from the library. While I came to enjoy having visitors, I also often found them annoying and fatiguing. I should have put a copy of the following passage from Miss Manners on my hospital door:

> *Patients' Behavior*
>
> There are considerable social advantages to being hospitalized, and it is too bad that most people who have the opportunity don't feel up to enjoying it. . . . Hospitalization . . . confers the official status necessary to legitimize errant behavior. The sick person with a healthy attitude will seize the chance. At no other time may you protect yourself so thoroughly from people you don't want to talk to or to see. From your birthday parties when your mother made you invite her friends' children you couldn't stand, right through the crowds of friends and spouses, spouses of friends, useful people and pitiful people, every other occasion has its share of people who can't be avoided. But not hospital life! You merely send word that you don't feel up to seeing anyone you don't want to see, or you get your doctor to do it.*

* * *

After a week in the hospital, I was worse. Much worse: white count down to 2,000 (normal is between 5,000 and 10,000); hematocrit, less than 30 (normal is between 37 and 47); hemoglobin, below 10 (normal is between 12 and 16); and platelet count *50,000*. Other tests regularly used to gauge the activity of lupus were also significantly abnormal, including the ANA (anti-nuclear antibody) test, a measure of the antibodies that attack the nuclear material of the body's own cells. While not a specific test for lupus (a positive ANA can be present in other diseases, or in the absence of disease), mine had been positive for years, usually at a titer of 1:320 or 1:640; but now it was 1:5120! The C-3 and C-4 complements are commonly measured to monitor lupus; normal values vary from lab to lab, but low complements generally indicate increased disease activity. At Lyman Memorial the normal ranges were 83 to 177 and 15 to 45, respectively. Now, my C-3 was down to 50 and my C-4 was 10. This was a very serious lupus flare, there

---

*Judith Martin, *Miss Manners' Guide to Excruciatingly Correct Behavior* (Atheneum, 1982).

was no more doubt about it—apparently precipitated by an otherwise ordinary respiratory infection.

Dr. Hoffman increased my Prednisone to 120 milligrams a day, in *four* divided doses. There seemed to be nothing else to do. Curiously, even this quantity of steroids—the ultimate anti-inflammatory drug—did not control my fever, and I continued to have temperature spikes up to 105 at least once a day. As if this was not absurd enough, one more inexplicable fact emerged. Only Tylenol kept my fever down! This oddity epitomized the entire situation. Nothing made any sense at all.

Dr. Hoffman came by that evening to tell me he was going on vacation for a week. I guess he needed it. Whatever was going on with me, my falling platelet count was the most immediate and most serious concern. So he was leaving Dr. Jones, the hematologist already involved in my case, in charge. The news made me feel abandoned. Dr. Hoffman *knew* me. I could *talk* to him. I could say anything to him, especially "NO." With Dr. Jones, I would have to be more deferential, more self-controlled. But he was a quiet, unassuming, gentle person. There was nothing about him not to like.

I settled in for the duration, more comfortable with my fevers controlled by round-the-clock Tylenol. Maybe I could just rest for a while and "enjoy" another weekend: visitors from the library; Scrabble at ten dollars a game with my father—the "house" bet; knitting, reading, watching television, writing letters. I was bored. I was restless. (Who wouldn't be on 120 milligrams of Prednisone?) Mostly, I was scared. Although no one had yet said anything to make me think so, I was beginning to wonder not *when* I would get over this episode, but *whether* I would get over it. The thought of dying didn't bother me as much as the uncertainty about what I would have to endure until then. And I didn't want to die in the hospital. It was good to have a week off to think about all this—a week off from having to put up a front for Dr. Hoffman.

Actually, Dr. Hoffman had ordered every conceivable test before he'd gone on vacation: a spinal tap (to rule out central nervous system infection); chest X-rays (to be sure I didn't have pneumonia); a sonogram and a CAT scan (I'm not sure for what); a gallium scan (to detect a hidden intra-abdominal infection); blood cultures; sinus X-rays; and a bone marrow (the most painful procedure I had ever endured, about which more later). Everything was negative.

I got off the IV, but continued taking antibiotics orally for the lingering respiratory infection. Nevertheless, my cough seemed to get worse, not better. I tried my best not to worry. I read novels I'd never had the time for. Anne Tyler. Edith Wharton. I sped up my knitting, finishing an entire baby blanket in one week. I caught up on some long overdue letters to friends I'd lost touch with over the years. I even wrote Eric— a clear sign I was trying to "put things in order." But there were many days when I couldn't do much at all, when I was too tired to do anything but listen to my pounding heart and feel the racing of my pulse as I tried to sleep. I didn't realize at the time that this was due to my progressive anemia, my heart and lungs working harder to oxygenate my tissues. Other times I was so agitated from the megadose of Prednisone—and the Actifed that had been added to my pharmacopoeia—that I could barely hold my hands still.

This medical crisis and my increasing recourse to the telephone for distraction helped to bring me and my sister closer together. Eva's call each evening became a part of the routine, like Dr. Hoffman's visit each morning. Both conversations soon focused on my platelet count. Each morning Dr. Hoffman would give me the number; each evening Eva would call and without so much as a "Hi, how are you," ask "How many platelets?" When Dr. Jones took over my case temporarily he looked puzzled when I told him I needed this information for my sister. He also thought it a little odd when my father kidded him that the only kind of bone marrow he cared about was the kind you *ate*.

On his last day in charge, Dr. Jones paused a long time before telling me that my platelets had dropped—*to 16,000*. The news made Eva pause even longer than usual. Or maybe silence is more dramatic over the telephone.

Eleven

It's not that I'm afraid to die. I just don't want to be there when it happens.
—Woody Allen

"That's about it, I suppose," I said to John and Karen, some two hours after I'd started to recount my life history.

They looked at me with a gaze I'd come to see often: a combination of disbelief ("you don't *look* like you have been so sick so long") and amazement ("you've handled it so well").

"Well, I don't eat alfalfa sprouts," I added to lighten up the mood. "I'll bet you didn't know they have been shown to aggravate lupus in monkeys. Now you may not think that's a problem, but you don't live where *I* do. Every time I go to a restaurant in Concord I have to tell them, 'Hold the sprouts.' And then they look at me like some anti-health food nut."

We all had a good laugh. Now I wanted to entertain them a bit more. "You know," I said to Karen, "I've always been annoyed at being told I couldn't get my ears pierced because of the possibility of infection. *Everyone* has pierced ears!" I stared enviously at hers. "Lately I've also been bothered when I'm mistaken for one of the students on campus. I suppose in another five or ten years I might appreciate the compliment, but not now. Being so short doesn't help. No one in my family is a giant, but I might have made it to five feet without all those early years on Prednisone. I even thought of putting streaks in my hair to look more sophisticated. But I read somewhere that the chemicals in hair colorings can aggravate lupus."

Alfalfa sprouts, pierced ears, streaked hair. It was insignificant, silly stuff. I thought about what I had just said—how in another five or ten years I might be glad to look younger than my true age. It dawned on me that all three of us wondered whether, for me, there would be another five or ten years.

Although the interview was fatiguing, I couldn't get to sleep after John and Karen left. I lay awake, thinking. Of course, much of what I had told them had gone through my mind before, but I'd never recounted the whole story to two strangers. I *had* been through a lot. I hadn't really given up anything that I now longed for. I felt at peace—contented with my life. I was prepared, intellectually and emotionally, to die. Some people might think I'm a fatalist. I prefer to consider myself a realist. Maybe I inherited what historian John Lukacs calls the "Magyar temperament," in which "a deep-rooted (and non-religious) pessimism is often broken by sudden bursts of appetite for life."

* * *

Monday, February 28. Dr. Hoffman returned from his vacation.

"Let's discontinue the Tylenol and watch your temperature. You can have some if it hits 40."

I was accustomed to reading both kinds of thermometers, so I knew that 40 centigrade equalled exactly 104 Fahrenheit. The new plan sounded like cruel and unusual punishment.

I had a restless night. By now I had a private duty nurse. This way I wasn't bothered by the nurses' scheduled routines for taking vital signs or giving me my "meds." Edna was a pleasant, elderly woman who didn't have to work too hard caring for me. I didn't need much— hot tea for the chills, ice bags for the fever, dry sheets and nightgown for the accompanying sweats. Perhaps it wasn't necessary for me to have my own nurse to bring me a snack at three a.m., but it did make me feel better. I've never figured out how Edna made an ordinary bowl of the instant oatmeal my father brought from home taste so much better than when I made it.

Tonight I wanted to walk the halls. I'd experienced lower back pain earlier in the evening. I thought if I kept walking, I'd walk it out. It was wishful thinking. Mysteriously overcome by severe abdominal cramps, I had to retreat from my hike around the sixth floor back to bed, begging for some pain killers. Edna succeeded, not without some difficulty, in getting me an order for one dose of codeine.

Morning came before the drug had enough time to take much effect.

I was still in intense pain; I hadn't slept a wink; I wasn't in the mood for morning rounds. With Dr. Hoffman, I could have a conversation. With some of the other doctors-on-rounds, *I* was an object *they* could converse about. The chief doctor would stand by my bedside, perform some perfunctory physical examination, summon one of his students to do the same, and then discuss the "findings" as if I were a cadaver.

One physician in particular grated on my nerves. I suspect the feeling was mutual. I'd crossed Dr. Fowler's path before, in 1980, when I was in Mansfield General. He was a rheumatologist I'd managed to avoid, a fact that could not have escaped his attention. As far as Dr. Fowler was concerned, he was a big cheese. As far as I was concerned, he was an outsider. I didn't want him meddling into my "case." One day, after he felt my cold hands, he explained to his pupils that this was a classic example of Raynaud's (common in lupus) and then turned to me and curtly suggested I put on a pair of gloves if I was uncomfortable. Brilliant. I was in no mood now for another of his intrusions. He did a cursory examination and pronounced his diagnosis: possible appendicitis.

When Dr. Hoffman arrived a short time later, I couldn't help but blurt out, "I don't ever want to see Dr. Fowler's face again! Can you *please* put a stop to his daily inspections?"

I didn't have appendicitis. I had a bad case of constipation, aggravated by the codeine. Dr. Fowler never came back.

Week three in the hospital began with Dr. Hoffman's decision to change my steroid medication from Prednisone to Medrol, the trade name for Methylprednisolone. I wondered what difference this would make. Was it merely a subtle way to increase the dosage? A hundred and twenty milligrams of Medrol was the equivalent of 150 milligrams of Prednisone. Dr. Hoffman also decided to administer the steroids in an IV drip, instead of by mouth. I didn't like the idea, or look forward to lugging the contraption around with me when I strolled the halls. It bothered me, most of all, for what it symbolized: how sick I really was, how much I really needed to be in the hospital. I began to understand what Flannery O'Connor meant when, shortly before she died, she wrote to a friend, "So far as I can see the medicine and the disease run neck and neck to kill you."

It was time for a second bone marrow. The first one had been bad enough. Not only had it been *my* first bone marrow, it was also the first for Dr. Jones's resident, Dr. Katz. I don't know which of us was more nervous. Dr. Jones stood there, in part to reassure me, in part to watch over his pupil. Lying on my stomach, face into my pillow, I could barely glimpse what Dr. Katz was doing. But I could see enough to notice a medieval looking drill just as he began to use it to grind a hole into the back side of my pelvis. This was one of those rare occasions when I would have preferred not being talked through the procedure, in all its detail. A shot of novocaine did deaden the pain, but the pressure of Dr. Katz's slow, methodical drilling was agonizing. Then he announced that he was extracting some fluid from inside— aspirating the marrow—to determine the cellularity. Was he talking to me? Or was he looking to Dr. Jones for approval? My interest in increasing my medical knowledge at this particular moment was nil. I could hardly move, much less carry on a conversation. So I grit my teeth and attempted to project a look of intense concentration in lieu of intense pain. What I needed most was some distraction. I told myself, surely I'd never have to endure a bone marrow again.

After less than forty-eight hours on the IV steroids, my platelet count rose to 70,000, not quite half of the low side of normal but a definite improvement. Maybe the Medrol was different; maybe the stuff was more effective in an IV drip. But none of the other serological tests showed even the slightest improvement. Nor did I feel any less tired, any less congested, any less disposed to near-constant coughing. I was also getting increasingly weaker, partly from bed rest, partly from steroid "myopathy"—the inevitable muscle wasting caused by the "treatment."

Within a few days, my platelet count had dropped again, down to 37,000. With my hematocrit below twenty, it was time for a blood transfusion, more specifically, a transfusion of "washed, packed, red cells." As the blood dripped into my veins, I could see the color in my hands turn from the palest white to the softest pink. The color change was accompanied by an equally instantaneous surge of energy. I could breathe more effortlessly; I could stroll the long corridors around *both* nurses' stations without stopping to take a break; I could stay awake to enjoy visitors.

I was glad I'd kept in touch with my old friend from Saint Maria's, Kate, and that she was still in town. She'd quit her job teaching junior high school English to pursue a PhD at Mansfield University. She had more free time now and lived only a few miles from Lyman Memorial. She could hardly believe how much better I looked, as she watched the transfusion create a transformation. We celebrated with extra large hot fudge sundaes. She was a real friend—someone who wouldn't let the sight of a large bag of blood interfere with good food.

Dr. Hoffman interrupted with an unusually late morning visit. He had a new plan.

"Your platelet counts haven't remained consistently above 50,000, even on the higher doses of Medrol. There's another method of steroid therapy, called pulse therapy. I think we should try it."

"Pulse therapy?" It sounded like "shock therapy." As it turned out, that wasn't far from the truth.

"Pulse steroid therapy means," Dr. Hoffman explained, "that we drip one gram of Methylprednisolone in one dose, once a day . . . on three consecutive days. Sometimes this 'jolts' the system, which not only brings an immediate improvement in the serological tests, but more important, sustains the improvement. I'd like to start that today. I don't anticipate any problems with it. But I can't say for sure it'll work."

I knew that went without saying. With a fresh supply of blood in my veins, I was feeling more agreeable than I had in weeks. Bizarre as the plan sounded, I couldn't see a reason to object.

When my father came by, as he did every day at lunchtime, I told him the latest news. He never imagined he'd use the tunnel connecting Mansfield General and Lyman Memorial so much. I could see in his eyes his reaction to the "pulse." But just as he shared my skepticism of the scheme, so also did he share my helpless acceptance of it. What else was there to do? There didn't seem to be much point in being in the hospital, with all its high tech procedures, if I was going to refuse them. And I wasn't ready to give up, yet.

Early that evening, the meds nurse came in with an armful of bottles, setting them up for the first of three pulse steroid treatments. I slept through the whole procedure, and awakened with a strange bitter taste in my mouth. When I reported this to Dr. Hoffman, he laughed it off. Weeks later, I got my hands on an article on pulse steroid therapy and discovered that this was one of its typical side effects! I was still a librarian first, a patient second.

The next morning, my platelet count was 59,000. It was too soon for the "pulse" to have any effect. I was ready for the second blast, scheduled for eight p.m., plenty of time for my after-dinner stroll through the halls.

No more than fifteen minutes after the drip was started, I began to feel a strange stiffness in my knees. I tried to move them, assuming that my legs had just "fallen asleep." That would explain the odd tingling as well. But it clearly wasn't that. When I pulled up my nightgown and saw two bright red knees, the color of well-cooked lobster claws, I was dumbfounded. And terrified. By now the pain was excruciating. I couldn't budge. I couldn't even reach for the call-button to summon a nurse. I screamed for help.

"I've never been in so much pain in my life!" I exclaimed as a nurse rushed into my room. "And look—my knees are BEET RED! What's happening?"

I didn't expect her to have an answer. And I certainly didn't expect her to say, "I don't know who I'm going to find on call tonight. All the residents are studying for the National Boards."

Luckily, before she ran out of my room in pursuit of a doctor she had the good sense to disobey *her* orders and turn off the steroid drip. This was the only intelligent, independent, decision I saw a nurse make during my entire hospital sojourn. It couldn't have come at a better time.

While she was gone, I managed, somehow, to reach the telephone at my bedside and call my father. He was still at Yinky's, eating dinner.

"You've got to come back here, NOW! I don't know what's happening. I can barely move. It started right after the drip. The nurse turned it off and she's trying to find a doctor. Maybe you should call Hoff at home?!" I hung up before my father had a chance to reply, surprised to see the nurse back so soon, and not alone. But when I took a good look at who was standing with her, I almost wished she had been.

I'd seen this face before. This guy had been a medical student or an intern, I didn't know which, three years before, when I was in Mansfield General with my alleged case of toxic shock. I remembered him as being arrogant and patronizing, and for taking a big, black magic marker to my body, circling the mysterious red spots on my chest, telling me, "I'll need to remember where they were, in case they fade or disappear." Then *he* disappeared. "What is he going to do to you *now*?" I thought to myself. My own look of horror was matched by his look of "Oh no, not *you* again."

Dr. Rubin had matured a lot in three years, thank God. Instead of lunging at me, armed to take some inappropriate action, he looked at the IV, checked to make sure it was shut off, turned to the nurse and said, matter of factly, "Where's Dr. Hoffman? Find him!"

My bad luck with the "pulse" was matched by my good luck in finding Dr. Hoffman on call that night. He was only a few floors downstairs in the hospital. Within minutes, both he and my father were standing in my room.

"Give her some Benadryl!" my father implored Dr. Hoffman as he took one look at the color of my skin. As usual, he did not hesitate to interject his own opinion. He assessed, correctly again, that I needed an antihistamine to counter this reaction, whatever the cause.

The next thing I knew, I was swallowing 50 milligrams of Benadryl, with 50 milligrams of Demerol for the pain. In half an hour, the color of my skin returned to its normal pale tone, and the pain began to dissipate. The combination of medications also made me extremely sleepy. I dozed off, unaware that the drip had been re-started.

I was barely awake, and far from "dressed," when Dr. Hoffman returned to my room in the morning.

"You had a pretty rough night last night. How are you now?"

"I'm glad you were here to see it. Otherwise I don't think you would have believed it! Do you have any idea what happened?" It all seemed like a bizarre nightmare.

"I'm not really sure. The solution may have been prepared too far ahead of time and settled, so the mixture wasn't correct by the time the drip was started. They don't do this very much around here." He seemed to be apologizing for the hospital's ineptitude, trying to demonstrate that it was an accident, not something inherently wrong with the procedure. How else would he get me to agree to the third treatment?

By the end of the week, my platelet count was up to 86,000. Maybe the blast was worth it. At least I had some hopeful news to get me through the weekend.

I had managed to persuade Dr. Hoffman to keep Dr. Fowler away from me. I didn't think I'd have to make a special plea about his resident. Completely unannounced—on a Sunday no less—he showed up in my room. A small, oriental man, about my own age. He could barely speak English.

"So, you have loopuss for lass twenty years?" he said as he walked through the door. No name. No stated purpose. Nothing.

"I'm only twenty-seven. I've had it since I was thirteen," I replied curtly. I wondered if anyone gets lupus at the age of seven.

"When you have flares before? What you feel?" he continued. Clumsily.

"Mostly joint pains, especially hands and knees, fatigue. I also had a bad skin rash subsequent to bug bites that wouldn't clear." It was all in my chart. Perhaps he couldn't *read* English either.

"So, you know your hemoglobins at those times?," he asked.

"How would I possibly remember *that*?" I was getting fed up, but could tell this guy wasn't finished.

"And how much more Prednisone you take with these flares?" Some question.

"That would depend on how much I was taking *before* the flare. Usually fifty percent more would be enough for a short period of time, and then I'd taper back down." As I guessed at the figure, I wondered if his math was any better than his English.

"Ever had same problem with your liver enzymes?"

Liver enzymes? Maybe he was in the wrong room. I didn't know what he was talking about.

He had no other questions. He only added how great Dr. Fowler was, how he was *always* right about "cases like mine," and concluded with a reassuring remark, "So, if pulse not work, that's all we do for you. Nothing else to do." Then he left.

There had been many times during the last month when I wished someone had come right out and said I might die. But this was definitely not what I had in mind. Clearly, Dr. Fowler had taught his residents to act just like him.

* * *

"I think it's time we start thinking about sending you home," Dr. Hoffman announced, first thing Monday morning. "Maybe Thursday." He paused. "Your platelet count seems to be dropping again. It's in the mid-fifties now. I'll take you off the IV, and start you on oral Medrol again, 20 milligrams four times a day, 80 total. And keep on with the Tylenol and Actifed as needed."

It was still hard for me to believe that only Tylenol controlled my fevers, and that I still needed a commonplace decongestant for my lingering respiratory symptoms.

"The latest films of your sinuses *did* show an infection," Dr. Hoffman continued. "So, I'm going to put you on Ampicillin as well, 500 milligrams, four times a day. You can take all this at the same time, to make it easier."

Very funny. I was taking *more* medicine than when I was admitted—and *now* I was about to be discharged?

"I guess the sinus infection proves I haven't been malingering all these weeks, huh?"

I laughed at my own joke. But I didn't think it was funny at all when Dr. Hoffman told me that one of the other physicians had seriously proposed just that as the diagnosis for what ailed me! He never told me who it was. I could guess.

Dr. Hoffman told me to start writing up a list of questions to ask him before my discharge. What could he possibly have in mind? Then it dawned on me that I had been allowed to do so little in the hospital, I really didn't know anymore what I *could* do when I got back home. Or what I *should* or should *not* do. I still remembered when Dr. Hauser had told me I could do whatever I felt up to doing. I doubted if Dr. Hoffman would be so permissive.

The rest of the day passed uneventfully, until Dr. Katz, the chief resident, arrived to announce, "I'm going to put an IV 'lock' in for your antibiotics."

Similar to a regular IV, into which a continuous drip can be placed, the "lock" is placed on the arm for periodic injections. It is less cumbersome than being permanently attached to a bag on a pole, but it's still a pain, literally and figuratively. At this point, it made absolutely no sense.

"Why should I get the antibiotics intravenously? I'm taking everything else orally now," I demanded. "Besides, Dr. Hoffman is planning to discharge me by the end of the week. I'll still be taking it then, and it won't be through an IV lock. So why now?"

"Because you are in the hospital now," he replied.

Logic didn't seem to be a required course in medical school.

Twelve

> Use your health, even to the point of wearing it out. That is what it is for. Spend all you have before you die; and do not outlive yourself.
> —George Bernard Shaw

Admission number 8884306. Date of admission: February 10, 1983. Date of discharge: March 17, 1983. I had endured more in these thirty-five days than in the previous fifteen years of living with lupus. And I had absolutely nothing positive to show for it. I was leaving the hospital not because I had improved, but because there was nothing more the doctors could do for me. The disease seemed completely out of control.

My father helped me pack my belongings: books, knitting, Scrabble game, stationery, cards and letters by the hundreds. I felt as though I were packing after a long vacation, having accumulated a hoard of junk I didn't have when I arrived. After saying my goodbyes to the nurses on Six North, I got the mandatory wheelchair ride and was taken down the elevator to my father's car. Although I was going home, I was more scared than the night I arrived at the emergency room by ambulance. The final diagnosis on my discharge summary read as follows:

> Fever of uncertain etiology;
> Thrombocytopenia, hypoplastic and destructive;
> Anemia, hypoplastic and destructive;
> Systemic lupus erythematosus;
> Sinusitis.

After five weeks of intensive scrutiny, the fever still had no known cause. And the thrombocytopenia and anemia were "destructive"—sufficiently plain English to say it all. "Thrombocytopenia" is the medical name for a low platelet count—now down to 34,000; "anemia" was the description for my hemoglobin of 9 and my hematocrit of 27, both terribly low. SLE, hardly something new. Sinusitis?—as if something so trivial, so ordinary, needed mentioning.

Finally, I was going home. I should have been overjoyed. But I was being discharged sicker than ever! I was terrified that something terrible would happen. I didn't know what. I knew how sick I was, how apparently hopeless my prognosis—even though no one actually said I was going home to die. The expression on Dr. Hoffman's face the morning of my discharge was, however inadvertently, eloquent.

I was discharged on 20 milligrams of Medrol, four times a day; 250 milligrams of ampicillin, four times a day; Actifed, four times a day; iron, three times a day; and folic acid, a member of the vitamin B complex group used in the treatment of anemia, once a day; plus periodic "shots" of Maalox. I made a chart to tape on the bathroom mirror to keep it all straight.

The short drive from Lyman Memorial was strenuous, but being outdoors, breathing the crisp air, was refreshing. Although I was very tired, I rarely slept very long, my steroid dose so high and so continuous it made me feel "wired." The Actifed further aggravated my agitation. To make matters worse, I was once again at Yinky's house, not my father's. I had no choice, for now. My father was at work during the day, and neither he nor I thought it would be wise for me to be alone. Staying with Yinky had to be better than the hospital. Unfortunately, sometimes I didn't think so.

Admittedly, I was unreasonable. But for five weeks I had tried not to behave as badly as I felt, to show the medical world how "well" I could look, how "well" I could sound, how "well" I could act. It was an *act*, all right. We all knew the truth, however little Dr. Hoffman said. Only my father and I discussed the truth straight out, in no uncertain terms. At Yinky's house, I still took the effort to "look well." But now I wanted to be able to *act* sick: I *had* to let down my guard. That meant admitting how sick I was, talking about it, complaining about it, and generally being insensitive to people around me—especially to anyone who pretended otherwise.

Because of her own anxiety about me, poor Yinky constantly fell into this trap. I would get angry at her for refusing to believe I probably would never get well, that I might soon die. She would get upset at being unable to help me. She just couldn't accept the truth. "Survivor guilt"? Probably. How could she watch her twenty-seven-year-old granddaughter deteriorate day by day, while she, just a few months short of *eighty-nine*, enjoyed miraculously good health and independence?

The first time I overheard her on the phone, telling one of her friends, "Oh, Suzy is much better," I went into a rage. "I am *not*! I am *NOT*!!" I screamed from the other room. Try as I might to convince her to tell the truth, she would repeat these clichés every chance she got. And the more often she did, the angrier I became. I know I should have shrugged it off. I couldn't change her ways. But I couldn't stand her "polite" lying. For me, *that* was worse than the truth.

I felt cooped up at Yinky's, but I didn't have the strength to go anywhere, and Dr. Hoffman had told me I shouldn't be out in public places because of my compromised immune system, enfeebled both by lupus and high doses of steroids. So movies or dinners at restaurants were out of the question. With winter still in full force, just driving around with my father was not particularly appealing. Better to stay inside and play Scrabble. At ten dollars a game, I was building up a sizeable bank balance. Hard as he tried, even with Scrabble dictionary in hand, my father rarely beat me. I wondered when, or if, I'd get the chance to spend the money.

After a few days I was pretty self-sufficient. I could take a shower by myself; fix myself something to eat; get whatever I needed. Then, one afternoon, hurrying to answer the telephone in the kitchen, I suddenly felt my legs buckling under me and tumbled to the ground. I assumed I'd tripped over one of Yinky's scattered oriental rugs. But when I tried to get up, I couldn't. I could barely lift my body up off the ground. My leg muscles were being destroyed by the Medrol: steroid myopathy, but good. I had to crawl to a chair and pull myself up. Even that was very difficult, the muscles in my arms having been greatly weakened too.

It was a rude awakening. I was confronted by a new fear: I was becoming *disabled*. Until now I had to deal only with being *diseased*, perhaps even terminally. That I had come to terms with. The prospect of being disabled was, to me, even more terrifying. Then I wondered if I'd live long enough to really have to worry about that prospect. The mind, my father loved to say, is an organ not for thinking but for rationalizing.

* * *

Tuesday, March 22. I hadn't seen Dr. Hoffman for five whole days.

"Your platelet count hasn't changed much. Yesterday's lab results showed it was 38,000. I think we should try cutting back on the Medrol. You can't stay on this dose. Let's go down to 16 milligrams, four times a day—64 milligrams a day."

I was so high into the megadose range of steroids that I couldn't see what difference this minor tinkering was going to make. But since the Medrol was clearly killing my muscles, and not helping my platelets as much as anyone hoped, this made some sense.

"The rest of the lab work looks about the same too," Dr. Hoffman continued, reading off only the numbers he knew interested me.

I left the office. Another week to kill before my next appointment, and not much hope for a change. My Medrol-euphoria aside, I was more tired than ever, napping every afternoon. This may have been the only habit I never acquired from my father. For me, this activity was completely out of character. Typically, I woke up only when my father arrived at Yinky's for dinner, feeling as though I'd been awakened from a sleep as deep as death. Day after day after day.

I was getting restless and found a new reason for my anxiety. I wasn't really at "home." I was at my grandmother's house. The more I thought about it, the more obsessed I became with the idea that this was why I still felt so lousy. I needed more privacy and space. I wanted to move to my father's house where I had my own bedroom. After five years of living on my own, it was still *my* room, everything kept the way it had always been. And it was much quieter in Thornden. It was outside the city, a beautiful, wooded suburb where the only noises were the occasional snowplow and woodpecker, soothing sounds compared to the constant dog barking and street traffic outside Yinky's house. But perhaps best of all, I could be home *alone* all day. My apprehension about being alone, so intense when I left the hospital, had lessened. Only at night was I a little fearful of "something happening." And at night my father would be home.

A week at my grandmother's house had been more than enough— for both of us. It was hard for her to deal with me. Too often she seemed not to take my illness seriously, exhibiting the denial typically found in the patient. At the same time, she took my behavior, which was admittedly callous and obnoxious at times, too seriously. I needed to express my feelings freely, without inner constraints. Yinky took my cathartic outbursts personally. We needed a separation. Better for me to yell at my father.

I decided to drive "home." No one had told me not to drive. I just hadn't felt up to it until now. I guess the anticipation of going to my father's house lifted my spirits. Besides, his house was ten miles from Mansfield. If this plan was going to work, I had to be able to drive myself to my medical appointments in town. Sitting behind the wheel of my own car for the first time in nearly two months, I revelled in my regained sense of independence. It was a typical cold, grey day. The lightly falling snow added a surreal beauty to the landscape without yet making the roads particularly dangerous.

I was HOME! The house was freezing cold, my father having turned the thermostat down to fifty-five when he left for work. With my temperature rising, the cool air was a welcome relief, especially after spending a week in Yinky's overheated house. I reset the dial to sixty-eight and walked about the house, exploring as if I hadn't seen it for years. I made a cup of tea and sat at the kitchen table, gazing out through the sliding glass doors onto the deck and the woods. Even through the misty grey air, I could see clear across the valley, through the leafless trees, the snow still falling. It was the first peaceful moment I'd had in weeks.

To get to my bedroom, I had to climb a flight of stairs. It was an ordinary dozen or so steps found in any standard, colonial-style house. I was glad I hadn't given this much thought before, or I might have chickened out and remained at Yinky's ranch-style house. I took one step at a time, holding tightly with both hands onto the wooden railing along the wall. When I finally made it to the top, I decided I'd had enough exercise for the day.

I slept through the entire afternoon, and woke up only when my father came home for dinner, the grinding sound of the electric garage door announcing his arrival. Although I slept soundly, my sensitivity to even small noises hadn't diminished. As usual, my father came upstairs to change before dinner. When I had lived at home years before I had often been annoyed by his unhurried evening ritual. I was always eager to eat the minute he walked through the door. Now I was grateful for his relaxed approach: taking out his false teeth (he'd had them since he was a young man, but they always bothered him); sipping Scotch; changing socks (his feet were always cold); putting on another suit he wore only at home. By the time he was ready, I was too.

"Why don't you go down first and wait at the bottom in case I topple over," I suggested at the top of the staircase.

My father gave me a look that said "maybe coming home wasn't such a good idea," but kept quiet, his forehead turning bright red, as if he were holding his breath. Actually, with the events in recent weeks, his forehead had taken on a permanently nervous-red hue.

"Don't get so EXCITED," I found myself shouting at him just the way I had been at Yinky. But he could take it. I started my way down, slowly, knowing that if I stumbled he might *really* get upset. I went down the way I went up, one step at a time, sideways, holding onto the railing with both hands. While it didn't take as much energy to go down as it did to go up, I felt as if I had to hold on carefully lest my legs cave in under me. Going up, I had to overcome gravity; coming down, I had to keep gravity from overcoming me.

It was the first evening of a new routine. I had always loved to cook and prided myself on doing it well. It was a talent I inherited from my mother.

"It looks like we're going to have to settle for tuna fish on English muffins," I announced, after a quick glance inside a nearly empty refrigerator. Thank God my uncle Andrew in Zurich always saw to it that there was a supply of Swiss chocolate in the house—dark, bittersweet truffles we called "balls." My father poured himself another Scotch and poured me an alcohol-free beer.

Without a doubt I was happier at my father's house. It was home. I had real privacy. And when I couldn't be alone, I preferred being with my father rather than my grandmother. Actually, she and I were similar on that score: She too preferred being with him than with me.

I had no idea how long I would be "home" and tried not to think about it. I didn't know where I was going next—to my apartment, to the hospital, or to my grave. I had no control over that. But I had to do something useful. While I've always liked to "veg out" for an afternoon, longer periods of inactivity are not my style.

The first thing my father and I had to do was make the house more manageable for me; the next thing was to make me feel more productive while I was stuck here. Going up and down the stairs any more than absolutely necessary seemed unwise. We certainly didn't need the formal dining room for entertaining. So we redesigned it as my "office." This way I could live on the first floor and go upstairs only to sleep and shower. We both cursed buying a house with no bedroom and full bathroom on the first floor, but it was too late for that.

I turned my energies, such as they were, to sorting out the medical bills and insurance forms I had amassed since my admission to the hospital. I looked through the piles, interested only in any medical bills that hadn't been paid by my insurance company. This required a good deal more patience and perseverance than brains, matching hospital and physician statements with those from Blue Cross/Blue Shield. I'd heard stories about strange items being charged to patients' hospital bills, and had been advised to check the bill for errors. I looked at mine: It was ten pages long, with undecipherable abbreviations for each service provided. I looked at the single-page statement from Blue Cross/Blue Shield, showing the balance of $15,487.00—paid in full. If there was an error, I didn't care. In fact, I found only one bill that wasn't 100 percent covered: the $135 charge for the ambulance to the emergency room. I should have taken a cab.

Then I recalled a more serious mistake I'd made, years ago, when I'd completely forgotten my extra medical insurance policies. At least I'd learned a lesson. It took hours to gather all the necessary information for my one-hundred-dollar-a-day In-Hospital Cash Plan. Thirty-five days. Thirty-five-hundred dollars! Tax free.

That out of the way, I settled down to my other homework. Dr. Hoffman had mentioned several remaining treatment options, and I wanted to read up on them. The two still being considered seriously were plasmapheresis and splenectomy. I sent my father out to the library at Mansfield General, and called my colleague and friend, Frank, at the library in Concord. Between the two of them, I knew I could get all the information I wanted.

I was vaguely familiar with the possible benefits and risks of splenectomy, the surgical removal of the spleen. Of course, the very idea of major abdominal surgery scared me. It brought to mind the joke, "The operation was a success, but the patient died." Even if my spleen was the cause of my platelet destruction—the main focus of attention now—and the splenectomy "worked," I didn't feel strong enough to withstand an operation.

Plasmapheresis was another matter altogether. It was mentioned only briefly in the most current textbook on lupus my father could find in the library,* which I had been reading for weeks now. Frank's computer search had turned up several articles, each one characterizing the treatment as highly experimental. Simply put, the procedure involved removing two to four liters of plasma—the non-cellular liquid portion of the blood—two or three times a week, and replacing it with another solution, usually human albumin. In theory, this therapy is supposed to cleanse the body of the excess immune complexes circulating through the system. It sounded like a ghoulish oil change to me, worse than the "pulse" treatment I'd undergone. At least the pulse required only three treatments over three days; plasmapheresis entailed a commitment to a series of treatments spread out over a longer period of time, taking longer still to assess the results. And, judging from what I was reading, the practical benefits sounded inconclusive, at best: "last-ditch measure," "has yet to be proved," "uncertain benefit," "transient improvement," "uncontrolled observations," "to be tried," "a preliminary report," were the phrases that caught my eye. They weren't very inspiring.

I read through some of the abstracts on Frank's computer printout. "After three months there was a severe relapse and the patient died"; "no significant changes . . . occurred"; "follow-up during the subsequent six months showed deterioration"; "plasmapheresis has an important role as a research tool." That did it—"an important *research tool*"!

Strangely, after hours of depressing reading, I felt much better. Although I had no definite plan about what to do next, I felt certain about what I did *not* want to do. I did not want to undergo a splenectomy just yet, and I did not want to undergo plasmapheresis at all. I rolled up the printout from the literature search, scanning through the especially ominous phrases now highlighted in red, and set it next to my purse so I wouldn't forget to take it to my next appointment with Dr. Hoffman.

* * *

Monday, March 28. Jill showed me right into Dr. Hoffman's office. She didn't want me to undress. That was not a good sign. It meant

---

*Schur, Peter, ed., *The Clinical Management of Systemic Lupus Erythematosus* (Grune & Stratton, 1983).

Dr. Hoffman wanted to have an earnest discussion, not examine me. As he walked in the room he seemed much more reserved than usual, the way he acted with my father, not me.

"Suzy, we have to start thinking seriously about the next option. You've been out of the hospital a week and a half now. Your lab work is unchanged. The only visible improvement seems to be a lessening of your respiratory symptoms, so you can stop the Ampicillin and Actifed." He went on, without a pause. "My major concern is the thrombocytopenia. You can't go on forever with platelet counts below 50,000. There are only a few possible therapies, some of which I've mentioned, but we haven't really talked about. There's plasmapheresis."

Politely, I interrupted him. I didn't want him to waste his time trying to sell me on that one. "Look, I know roughly what it is. I don't like it. Here." I handed him my annotated references on the subject. I may have been losing platelets, but I hadn't lost any brain cells. Sixty-four milligrams of Medrol a day also helped me sound stronger than I really was. "Got any other ideas?"

"We could increase the Medrol—drastically—and see if that boosts your numbers. We can explore the merits of splenectomy, or . . ." he paused and looked straight at me, "you could go to the National Institutes of Health in Bethesda, Maryland, and see Dr. Lowell for an evaluation. He's had a patient with a case remarkably similar to yours who is doing very well after splenectomy. I really think *that's* what you should do."

I could feel tears welling up in my eyes. I felt crushed. I could hardly speak. "But I don't feel well enough for surgery. I'm still coughing. All I want to do is sleep. I need more time."

Dr. Hoffman's eyes said, "You don't have all the time in the world." He, too, seemed about to lose his cool. "Well," he went on, "you can try *doubling* the Medrol, to 128 milligrams a day. But if you don't respond very quickly, you really ought to go to NIH." Then, as a desperate afterthought, he added, "If you were *my* daughter, I'd *send* you to NIH!"

If that was supposed to tell me he really cared, it didn't work. I knew he cared. Now, I felt that he wanted to get rid of me, that he didn't want me to die in his care. Then he could tell himself, and everyone else, that he had tried everything. But I had been through the go-see-the-experts routine before, in 1980. And while the present situation was far more serious, it was also more simple. Dr. Hoffman had already gone over *every* detail of my case with Dr. Lowell over the telephone. He himself had told me that. And Dr. Lowell had already given his recommendation—splenectomy. So what else could he do, except see me, face to face?

"Look," my voice began to crack, "I was *born* in Bethesda. I don't want to *die* there!"

I was born at the National Naval Medical Center while my father was on active duty as a commander in the Navy. My mother liked to tell the story that when the two of them were in line together at the supermarket—my father dressed in uniform complete with cap adorned with "scrambled eggs"—the cashier, overhearing their conversation (and my father's thick accent) asked my mother politely, "Which Navy is your husband serving with, ma'am?"

I was not joking, and Dr. Hoffman knew it. "Okay, we won't talk about NIH anymore . . . today. The splenectomy option won't run away. It sounds like you'd rather try increasing the Medrol for now, right?"

Actually, I would have preferred to do nothing—and die. But I decided to keep my mouth shut for a change, and nodded in agreement instead. I could "do nothing" later. It was a hard session for both of us. I looked up at Dr. Hoffman for some final words of wisdom. None came. His usual pat on the shoulder, this time nearly a hug, was the best he could do.

Dr. Hoffman and I had never been so seriously at odds before. But the more I thought about it, the more I knew I was right about NIH. There was nothing to be gained from going there, and much to be lost—especially whatever little control I still had over my fate. There, the balance of power between doctor and patient would be tilted hopelessly in favor of the doctor. The medical establishment at NIH would broach no disagreement, playing on their own home turf.

The conversation over dinner with my father was, as usual, brutally frank. "A HUNDRED AND TWENTY EIGHT milligrams of Medrol?" The speed of my father's voice escalated with each word. He was incredulous and upset.

I waited until he was on his second glass of Johnny Walker Black before pointing out to him that 128 milligrams of Medrol was the equivalent of *160* milligrams of Prednisone. This may have been the only medical detail I knew better than he.

"What about your bones? What about your muscles? For how long?"

My father's questions were a cascading torrent. I could hardly stop him.

"Wait a second," I interjected, trying to put him in my shoes. "It was either this or plasmapheresis or splenectomy or a trip to NIH. We already agreed the plasma thing is out, and we're both ambivalent about the splenectomy. When Hoff hit me by surprise with the NIH proposal, I just about lost it. I told him I was born there and I didn't want to die there." The line hadn't made Dr. Hoffman laugh, but it broke through my father's frown.

"You didn't say *that*, did you?" He was obviously pleased with the retort. I could tell I'd inherited my father's wicked sense of humor.

"Don't the doctors at NIH know all about your case already? What do they need to *see* you for? Why don't you tell Hoff I'll send them a *photo* of you instead!" Now my father laughed out loud.

After three ultra-megadoses of Medrol—before twenty-four hours had elapsed—I noticed a side effect: I barely napped, never mind slept. Before, I felt "wired"; now I felt the wire was about to snap. But one could get used to this high, I thought to myself. I was glad for the extra "energy" as I readied myself for another trip into town, an appointment with my ophthalmologist, Dr. Drysdale. He wasn't just the first doctor I went to. He was my favorite.

"You're looking better than when I saw you in the hospital, Suzabelle." He had called me that ever since I'd met him, more than twenty years before. Knowing him as long as I had, I found this diminutive—even at the age of twenty-seven—endearing, not at all a put-down.

"Actually, I do *feel* better. Thanks, again, for visiting me in the hospital. It was one of the few nice surprise visits I received. Things are about the same, blood-wise. Dr. Hoffman and I decided to increase the steroids, to 128 milligrams of Medrol a day. We're hoping my platelet count will rise and stay there."

Dr. Drysdale looked aghast. I began to have second thoughts myself about this new plan when he informed me that the high doses of steroids I'd been taking since late January had already affected the muscles in my eyes—so much so that I needed a new refraction for my eyeglasses. Nothing very alarming, yet, but my eye muscles were showing signs of weakness—like the muscles in my arms and legs. Although he didn't say so, I knew he was even more concerned about the other potential hazards of this absurd regimen: cataracts and glaucoma. I tried to reassure him—and myself.

"I don't think I'll stay on this much Medrol very long. I'm seeing Dr. Hoffman every week now. The plans keep changing. I'll keep you posted."

"I'd like to see you in three months, instead of your usual six."

Three months. I could only think in terms of days. I returned home, and was about to call Dr. Hoffman when the phone rang.

"I've got a new plan," he announced, sounding upbeat.

I was surprised to hear from him so soon. New plan? The old one had only been in effect twenty-four hours.

"I want you to see Dr. Ernst on Monday. He's at the Hematology Clinic at Mansfield General. He'll do another bone marrow, and some other platelet studies. But before that, I've scheduled you for a bone marrow scan in Nuclear Medicine, for Friday, at one o'clock. You should probably go with your father. They may not want you to drive home afterwards."

Not drive? What were they going to scan me with? "Where do we go after that?" I asked, puzzled by the news.

"I'll talk to Dr. Ernst after he sees you. I want his opinion about a splenectomy in your case. Get some rest, and make an appointment with Jill for a week from Friday, the eighth."

Rest seemed impossible, in my speeded-up state. "What about the Medrol? Keep it at 128?"

"Until the eighth . . . then we'll see."

Undergoing a splenectomy still sounded like a bad idea to me, no matter who he'd found in town who thought otherwise. The literature certainly wasn't inspiring. I scanned through the few articles my father had retrieved from the library, but which I thought I'd never have to read: "A Critical Look at the Splenectomy—SLE Controversy," "Splenectomy for Hemocytopenia in Systemic Lupus Erythematosus," "The Role of Splenectomy in the Treatment of Thrombocytopenia Purpura Due to Systemic Lupus Erythematosus," "Thrombocytopenia in a Young Woman." The last one caught my attention first.

"A fifteen-year-old girl was admitted to Barnes Hospital . . . because of thrombocytopenia. She died twenty-three days later." Great. I read on, feeling as if I were reading my own case history: She had also experienced a viral infection, low platelet counts, packed red blood cell transfusions, and high-dose Prednisone therapy. Her story sounded a little better than mine because her temperature had remained normal. But, buried deep within the article, were a few positive lines.

> The majority of patients cannot be managed adequately by steroid therapy alone; either they fail to respond entirely or they require so much steroid for maintenance that toxicity becomes a serious problem. Such patients usually come to splenectomy. Of splenectomized patients, about 70 to 80 per cent will be greatly benefited and many appear to be "cured."

I realized that this author was addressing the effect of splenectomy on thrombocytopenia alone, leaving its effects on lupus in limbo. I searched for something more pertinent. What there was, was not encouraging.

> Little information is available to the surgeon who is asked to evaluate for possible splenectomy a patient with thrombocytopenia purpura due to systemic lupus erythematosus. . . . Splenectomy should be reserved for those patients in whom steroid therapy is ineffective. . . . On the other hand, patients who represent a high surgical risk because of widespread lupus or other medical problems should be maintained on corticosteroids.

I was long past a three-to-four week trial period of high-dose steroids, never mind that these authors considered *forty* milligrams of steroids a day a high dose! But wasn't I a "high surgical risk"? Their concluding recommendation was useful, but worrisome.

> We advise against maintaining good risk patients on high dose steroids for a prolonged period of time in the vain hope of avoiding an operation. This attitude subjects those patients to complications of steroid therapy that are worse than SLE itself if the major clinical problem is thrombocytopenia.

Perhaps splenectomy was the right course. There was no denying my progressive muscle weakness. By now I couldn't even get up from the dining room table without firmly grasping the arms of my chair in order to push myself up. I should have stopped reading, but turned to one last article that seemed to offer another positive note. "Splenectomy is done frequently in patients with systemic lupus erythematosus." The pages that followed quickly demolished my hopes:

Besides the risks and morbidity of an operative procedure such as splenectomy, our study shows that splenectomy provides no long-term benefit better than medical treatment in the management of SLE patients with thrombocytopenia purpura or hemolytic anemia. Furthermore, there were more infections, more cutaneous vasculitis, and more deaths among SLE patients subjected to splenectomy than in the control group of patients treated medically.

I had always believed that information was power. Now, it only confirmed my powerlessness over this disease—and, seemingly, over what to do.

Thirteen

> Even if the doctor does not give you a year, even if he hesitates about a month, make one brave push and see what can be accomplished in a week.
> —Robert Louis Stevenson

Friday, April 1. I wanted to take a nap as soon as I'd finished breakfast, my muscular fatigue overtaking my wired state. I didn't have the strength to tackle the stairs, so I settled for the living room sofa with its deep, soft, comfortable cushions. I felt as though I'd dropped into a cloud.

I dozed all morning and awoke fully only to the sound of the electric garage door. My father had returned home to drive me to Mansfield General for my bone marrow scan. I tried to get up from the sofa, but couldn't, my rear end glued to the pillows.

"DADDY!" I shouted, before he was half-way in the house. "I CAN'T GET UP!" I cried, in horror and disbelief. As my father put his arms around my waist to help lift me, the odd sensation of feeling like dead weight remained.

Instead of saying something sympathetic, my father couldn't control his own emotions: "Don't you see . . . you can't stay on this much Medrol. Look what it's doing to your muscles. Imagine what it's doing to your *bones*. You just can't *feel* that yet." I knew he'd been waiting to say this for days, if not weeks. His sense of frustration was reaching its outermost limits.

I packed a few items for the trip into town: a book, knitting, the drugs I needed for the rest of the day. I was always prepared for long waits. My father and I shared the longest half-hour drive, ever.

Even holding onto my father's arm, the walk from the car to the hospital entrance was difficult and exhausting. Nuclear Medicine was in the basement. The very term "nuclear medicine" sounded mysterious to me. We got off the elevator. There were no people in sight. Just a lot of closed doors with skull and crossbones warnings posted on the outside: Danger! Radiation! Finally, at the end of a long corridor, we came to a waiting-room. Patients. Technicians. A receptionist who was unusually friendly.

"You must be Mrs. Szasz. You're having a bone marrow scan?"

It was such a pleasant surprise to be greeted so politely, I felt petty correcting her, "Yes, but it's *Miss*."

"The resident will be with you shortly to explain the procedure," she said, handing me a clipboard with a questionnaire to complete.

I looked around. It seemed to me that most of the patients were at the end of their ropes. When they left for home, it probably wasn't for long. Did this explain the kid-glove treatment? It was a depressing thought. Better just to be grateful for being treated decently.

"Hello. My name is Dr. Randolph. I'm going to do the bone marrow scan. Has anyone explained this to you . . . and your father?" he said, acknowledging *both* of us.

"I had a gallium scan last month. I guess it's something like that, right? You're trying to determine how my bone marrow is functioning in order to evaluate the merits of undergoing a splenectomy."

Dr. Randolph, who was about my age, continued patiently with his explanation. "It's similar, but this time you'll get a radioactive injection instead of drinking a radioactive liquid. Then we'll have you lie down on a table, while the scanner moves back and forth across your body, recording, by means of photographic images, the areas where the radioactive substance remains deposited. The procedure allows us to ascertain how actively your bone marrow is functioning. We need to determine whether your body is producing platelets normally but destroying them just as rapidly, or not producing them properly to begin with."

Dr. Randolph didn't mention splenectomy, but I knew it would be viable only if the former proved to be the case. It was troublesome, then, for me to feel hopeful about the outcome of the bone marrow scan when a favorable result would *support* undergoing a splenectomy— an option that still frightened me—and an unfavorable result would *destroy* that option altogether. Either way, I seemed to lose.

"Susan," Dr. Randolph concluded, "I have to ask you to sign a release form to show that you understand the procedure and its side effects. This is required—and I should tell you that we haven't experienced *any* problems—because the substance we use in the injection has only limited approval by the FDA."

"What kind of side effects are we talking about?" I asked, thinking of a TV melodrama, the doctor telling the patient about the possibilities of paralysis or blindness or permanent disfigurement.

"Well," he paused, "you could get a high fever for a couple of hours afterwards. You might want to rest here a bit when we are all through before you go home."

At that very moment, my temperature was at least 101. I barely had time to glance over at my father when we both broke out into laughter at the words "high fever."

"Let's get this glow-in-the-dark show over with," I said to a startled Dr. Randolph.

The results of the scan wouldn't be known until the following Monday. There wasn't much point in thinking about it before then. On the way home from the hospital, my father and I stopped off at Yinky's for dinner. We hadn't been there since I'd moved out. Now that she and I had enjoyed a week's separation, we could enjoy each other's company again. And the food! Maybe it tasted especially good because I didn't have to cook it. The chicken paprikas, swimming in rust-colored sour cream, would have tasted even better with a cold beer. I wondered if I'd ever be permitted to drink again.

I decided to take advantage of the good mood. "If the weather cooperates, can we go to Concord tomorrow?" I asked my father, hardly believing I dared. "Don't get excited," I continued, "I don't intend to make this a social gathering. I won't tell *any* of my friends I'm coming. I just need some more things from my apartment and it would be too complicated to tell you exactly what. I feel well enough. It's only an hour, you know."

My father readily agreed. Maybe he thought it wasn't such a wild idea. Or maybe he thought it was, but didn't have the heart to say no.

Why did I want to go to my apartment? It was obvious that I was likely to remain at my father's house for some time. There were only six weeks left of the spring semester at the university. There was no way I would see the library again before the end of this term. The logic of the work schedule suggested waiting until the middle of the summer, or even the beginning of the fall semester before returning, another three to six months, at best. Actually, I had the feeling that I wasn't going to return permanently to my apartment, or to the library—*ever*. That's why I wanted to bring more of my belongings to my father's house.

I needed some of my files for my insurance paperwork. I wanted my own electric typewriter instead of having to use my father's ancient manual machine. I could use more of the yarn I had stockpiled to start some new projects. But my father could have retrieved all those items by himself. What I wanted were things I wouldn't want to write down on a list. Even if I did, probably only I could find them: an album of photos from the family trip to Budapest, my favorite sheepskin slippers, a worn camel hair sweater, an onyx necklace from Eric, some Gordon Lightfoot records. I had considered myself extremely fortunate that I felt so at home—existentially, spiritually, mentally—at my father's. These few material objects were all that was missing.

My pessimistic agenda aside, the trip and the brief change of scenery lifted my spirits. By Monday morning I was ready for my appointment with Dr. Ernst. For some inexplicable reason, I even felt hopeful. Resigned.

Dr. Ernst was a large, loud man, younger, I suspected, than he looked. He talked faster than anyone I knew, with the possible exception of my father. Clearly he was interested in both me and my "case." There was an air about him of the wild-eyed scientist embarking on a major experiment that made me a little nervous. But he spoke to me with genuine concern, even affection, as if he had known me personally for a long time.

"I've heard a lot about you from Dr. Hoffman," Dr. Ernst introduced himself. "Don't worry . . . only good things!"

I suddenly felt as though I had a reputation to uphold. Well, I had earned the Model Patient Award the hard way. Why shouldn't I reap some benefits from it?

"My colleague, Dr. Alexander, is going to take a brief history, do a physical, and then perform a bone marrow. I know you had that done in the hospital, so you know what to expect," Dr. Ernst added.

I undressed for the most painful procedure I have ever undergone. At least I no longer suffered from fear of the unknown. But this time, when I attempted to lift myself up onto the examining table, I discovered I couldn't do it alone. Dr. Alexander, who had briefly left the room, returned to find me still standing by the table.

"Can you give me a hand, please?" I didn't have to say why.

Once horizontal, I lay on my stomach for the biopsy. Head on the pillow, I wanted to doze off, but Dr. Alexander continued to chat.

"First I'll give you an injection of novocaine. That will sting a bit."

Sting a bit? Nothing compared to the agonizing pain that would follow. But before I knew it, Dr. Alexander was done. Not with the injection, with the whole procedure! I had barely felt anything. This, I had to conclude, was the difference between a novice and a master: not just to be quick, but, more important, to be sure of oneself.

Dr. Alexander complimented me on my cooperativeness, but added, "You know, one of the reasons this was so easy, besides your being such a good patient, is because . . . your bones are like mashed potatoes."

I had no time to contemplate what he was saying before Dr. Ernst came flying back into the room. He launched into an explanation of the possible results of the bone marrow. I'd never heard so much detail so quickly in my life. There was no way I could keep up with him. But his conclusion was clear.

"If the results today are similar to the earlier biopsies and consistent with the bone marrow scan, then a splenectomy is in order. It looks like you definitely have an *active bone marrow*, with high cellular levels, and that the platelet destruction is taking place in the spleen. Removing it should reverse the thrombocytopenia. You'll be off the steroids in no time!"

I liked Dr. Ernst. I was ready to be convinced. I wanted to be convinced. But paradoxically, the more excited he became, the more skeptical I became. I could accept that the splenectomy might cure the thrombocytopenia, but what about the lupus? Dr. Ernst didn't seem to want to consider the possibility that the cure for one condition might, in fact, aggravate the course of the other. The suggestion that I might get off steroids *completely*, after fifteen years, seemed absurd—so wild it made me wonder how good Dr. Ernst's judgment was about the thrombocytopenia. Could he really be right? I was torn between wanting to believe him and not wanting to get caught up by false hopes. Dr. Ernst was obviously deeply concerned. He was an irresistibly lovable man, sure of himself but without a trace of pretentiousness, and truly caring.

* * *

I was always prepared for bad news from Dr. Hoffman, especially in recent weeks, about *me*, that is. I readied myself for today's account.

"Dr. Ernst has had a heart attack!"

I was shocked. Luckily, he was doing fine, so well, in fact, that he continued to badger Dr. Hoffman about me and the splenectomy from his hospital bed! Poor Dr. Hoffman. Now he had the patient's doctor for a patient as well.

"Dr. Ernst reviewed the results of your bone marrows and the scan along with your latest lab work. And, no, that's not what gave him a heart attack! He definitely thinks you should have a splenectomy."

"So I was right about NIH!"

It was all I could think to say. Anyway, it was true. And it wasn't meant to undercut Dr. Hoffman. On the contrary, it was meant to show him there were enough competent and caring doctors right here in town.

Dr. Hoffman continued to explain, in more amusing detail than before, just what was happening to my blood: "Your bone marrow is 25 to 30 percent cellular, which is good. And your reticulocyte count is well within the normal range. That means you are making plenty of new red blood cells. But then they are being destroyed. Like a game of Pac-Man . . . red cells being gobbled up as soon as they appear."

It was the first time in weeks we both laughed.

Dr. Hoffman ended our meeting with a vague and somewhat disconcerting conclusion. "Of course, your next appointment with Dr. Ernst has been cancelled. Let's lower the Medrol to 80 milligrams a day. And I want you to have a blood transfusion on Monday, the usual lab work on Wednesday, and I'll see you here next Friday, a week from today. We'll see where we stand then. Okay?"

I spent the weekend reflecting about my life. What was happening to me? I had already made some important, terrifying decisions—to take an absurd amount of steroids, to reject plasmapheresis, to refuse to go to NIH. Yet, at the same time, I felt I was, more or less, just going along with the flow. Now I was faced with what seemed like a truly ultimate and unavoidable choice: to go ahead with the splenectomy—knowing the possibility that not only might it do no good, but might even hasten my death, or to refuse the splenectomy and slowly return to an "acceptable" steroid dose—knowing the virtual certainty of further deterioration due to the steroids plus lupus complications, and death.

Actually, I was now convinced that I would die—no matter what I did. So I began to think not about whether I would die, but how I would die, and how I *wanted* to die. The options seemed clear: a slow, perhaps painful death if I chose to refuse further treatments (including more blood transfusions) and continue on steroids alone, or a quick, painless death if I chose to go ahead with the surgery and died on the operating table, or perhaps something in between, like dying from pneumonia or some other post-operative complication.

I found myself considering the splenectomy more favorably, but not for the same reasons Dr. Hoffman or Dr. Ernst did. They liked the idea because they thought it would cure me. I liked it because I thought it would kill me, quickly and painlessly.

My father accompanied me to the lab on Wednesday, not because I couldn't manage alone, but because we were also going to visit Dr. Ernst. This had to be the strangest doctor-patient-doctor arrangement ever. So there we were—me, my father, Dr. Ernst—conferring in a hospital room in Lyman Memorial. But the staging was all wrong. The doctor was lying in bed and the patient was sitting at his side, and neither of us looked sick. Aside from the hospital bed and gown, he looked exactly the same as the last time we'd met, just as feisty, and talking just as fast and just as optimistically.

"You're looking much better, Suzy. The results of the marrows and the scan confirmed everything. There's no question about the splenectomy . . . and you'll be off the steroids completely before you know it." He was flying, again.

By this time, his excessive enthusiasm was thoroughly endearing. I was ready to go along with the idea now, even though I didn't think it was going to "work," so it made no difference if I thought his opinion about the long-term prognosis of my lupus was wildly unrealistic. I could sense that my father was just about to put in his own two cents and muffle Dr. Ernst's zeal, but I gave him a "don't bother, there's no point" stare. Why spoil Dr. Ernst's eagerness? Especially now. He wasn't feeling so great himself. If seeing me and the prospect of my being "cured" by his recommendation made him feel better, why put a damper on it? Even in bad health, he was a doctor who cared as much about his patients as himself, maybe more.

In any case, our discussion was cut short with the arrival of Dr.

Ernst's lunch, an appropriate time to leave. As we said our goodbyes, he took a badly overcooked baked potato from his tray and flung it across the room.

"How's anyone supposed to eat this shit!" he shouted at the nurse, just missing her. "You could kill someone with one of these."

What a man!

* * *

My father's birthday, income tax day, was just two days away. I hadn't forgotten. But what could I possibly do for him? Only one thing came to mind: I would surprise him and finish editing the paper he'd given me to work on. I had initially resisted his request. I wasn't that interested in the subject—the Berkeley initiative to ban ECT (electroconvulsive therapy). I thought his draft was much too rough. It needed less psychiatry and more political philosophy. I knew I could improve his argument, but I insisted I was too sick. He rejected all my protests. He'd heard them before and insisted they were not valid excuses. He was right. But so was I.

My father's unfinished writing project reminded me of one of my own. I needed to write my will. I didn't neglect it because I had avoided the subject of dying. On the contrary. At home, my father and I had talked about it frequently, so much so, I became unconcerned about the legalities. They would be my father's problems, not mine! He *knew* what was important to me, what I would want him to do: that I didn't share his preference for cremation over burial, that I wanted some mildly religious service, that Kate, my good Catholic friend, would help him with that (and she knew she would too), that I wanted music, Albinoni's "Adagio for organ and strings in G minor" and Simon and Garfunkel's "April Come She Will" (I didn't care that this was an odd combination), that I wanted Eva to have all my clothes, and the library to have all of my money. It seemed unnecessary to put it all in writing. Or was it that doing so would make it *real*?

Talking about dying was easier than writing about it, but only with my father. No one else wanted to talk about it. I couldn't discuss my prognosis with my friends from work. My colleagues at the library tended to make the hour-long drive from Concord to Thornden in groups, making the occasions into pleasant, but often superficial, social calls.

I soon realized that I could count on one hand the number of friends who really knew how I felt, who really knew—or cared to know—exactly what was going on. There was Kate, who lived in town, had seen the worst in recent weeks-turned-months, and had known me the longest; Christine, my best out-of-town friend, who was used to commiserating with me, ever since we met at the television station and realized how overeducated we were for our jobs, and with whom it was easy to talk, perhaps because it was never face to face; Jackie, who worked in a different library at the university in Concord and managed to make the extra effort to visit me by herself, even if she didn't come as often; Jeff, one of the thousands of students I'd met across the reference desk who everyone said had a terrible crush on me, who called constantly, and was strong enough to ask, "You *are* going to get better, *aren't* you?"—and accept "I doubt it" for an answer; and Frank, who *had* to know, without asking, from all the literature he was sending me.

I realized, eventually, that I had to stop trying to talk about my dying. Death and dying were taboo subjects for everyone except my father.

* * *

Another week passed, and my platelet count held its own. My muscles remained very weak. I persuaded Dr. Hoffman to let me go to Lyman Memorial as an outpatient for physical therapy. Someone should have thought of this *weeks* before. It gave me a chance to get out of the house, provided some structure to my daily activities, and held out some promise of slowing down the steroid-induced muscle deterioration.

Outpatient P.T. turned out to be a happy choice. Carol, the physical therapist assigned to me, and I hit it off right from the beginning. She was about my age and not much bigger. But she certainly was stronger. I liked the way she pushed me to work hard, yet knew exactly when to stop before I would hurt myself or give up in frustration. I quickly learned to trust her, despite a few minor disasters.

The first occurred during our very first session, an evaluation to assess how much strength I had, or didn't have, and determine which muscle groups needed special attention. Carol decided to put me on the parallel bars, where I was to hold on and take deep knee bends.

But even before she had a chance to step away and attend to another patient, I took my first bend down, and landed flat on the floor. I couldn't get up. Fortunately, there were plenty of people in the room to help. It took three therapists to lift my light but completely limp body back to an upright position.

Carol looked startled, but her teasing cheered me up: "Susan, you're such a *noodle*!"

Sitting in a chair doing leg lifts was hard work. With a five-pound weight around my ankle, I couldn't budge my foot. Carol seemed surprised. I guess I didn't look so weak, just like I didn't look so sick. Better to start with one pound for the time being. More leg lifts, on my back, on my belly. Next, I stood on my tiptoes and walked in a straight line. Not-so-fond memories of a strict ballet teacher flashed through my mind. Then I tried to walk on my heels. It seemed utterly impossible. I wondered if I had *ever* been able to do this.

Carol began spending more time with me doing "resistance exercises," pushing and pulling my arms and legs. I think she enjoyed the opportunity to treat a patient with whom she could also talk. Sadly, many of the patients in P.T. were old, nearly comatose bodies who responded to the therapists' promptings with moans and groans if they responded at all.

When I told Carol I'd been ice skating just three months before, she looked at me in disbelief. I tried to explain how I used to be able to do a camel spin and a half-flip. And how at each figure skating club recital, *I* was chosen to be the girl to chase the pinwheel because I was the shortest—and could run fastest across the ice on my toe-picks. It was the only occasion I liked being so short. In just weeks all that skill, coordination, and strength had vanished. As I struggled with each step on the rung of practice-stairs, I couldn't believe I'd ever been able to spin or jump or stand up straight on ice.

By the end of April, despite the steady cutbacks in my steroids and the more intense physical therapy—now one hour, three times a week—I had become progressively weaker. Much weaker. Stairs were almost non-negotiable, sitting up in bed was a struggle, getting up from the toilet was, literally, a pain in the ass. I was beginning to doubt if the steroid myopathy was reversible, as I'd been told. Also, I was starting to feel more achy and feverish again. After several weeks of near-normal temperatures, without Tylenol, I unexpectedly had a fever spiking over 103. My lab tests deteriorated: white count, 2,000; hemoglobin, 10; hematocrit, 29; platelets, 43,000. The blood transfusion hadn't sustained my red count for long; the experimental course of high dose Medrol had failed to sustain even a near normal platelet count. I knew from the numbers that I had reached the end of the road. Now it was splenectomy—or nothing. I felt as though I'd been read my last rites.

"I guess," I said hesitantly to Dr. Hoffman at my next appointment, "it's time for the splenectomy."

Dr. Hoffman looked more relieved than pleased. Did he want me to have the splenectomy because he believed it would work or because he believed we had to do *something*? He didn't know that I agreed because I believed it would end my suffering quickly and painlessly.

"I'll make an appointment for you to see Dr. Cheever, the surgeon, next week," Dr. Hoffman responded, reassuringly. Obviously, he already had someone lined up.

As usual, my father and I talked at length over dinner that night. He seemed to accept my decision in much the same frame of mind as I had. There really wasn't any other choice left. The alternative was a certain, slow, death. It was time to break the news to my sister and brother-in-law. Eva and Michael were unenthusiastic about the splenectomy from the beginning. Why? Because its value was not supported by the literature, because I was a poor surgical risk, and perhaps because it wasn't their idea. Actually, they also thought it would kill me. Maybe it was just as well they were so far away. All I could do was make faces they couldn't see, and point out that they had no better suggestions to offer. It was a desperate situation for them, too. But with Eva and Michael I had to pretend that I had more faith in the splenectomy than I did, feeling that I had to justify myself—medically, not existentially.

And then there was Yinky. She was easy. Being ever ready to refuse to accept that I was so desperately ill, she was the most willing to blindly believe that what was wrong with me could be "fixed."

My father and I went to see Dr. Cheever together. I'd never been in a surgeon's office before. It looked unlike any other doctor's office I'd ever seen: smaller, *much* more elegantly furnished, fewer people waiting. We were ushered into a small conference room as soon as we arrived. It was not an examining room. There wasn't anything to examine, of course. I was way past that.

"Dr. Cheever will be right in. Can I get either of you a cup of coffee?" the secretary/nurse—it was hard to tell which—inquired, as she turned to leave the room. I felt as though I was in a lawyer or stockbroker's office, waiting to discuss my divorce or stock portfolio.

Dr. Cheever's appearance and demeanor completed this businesslike atmosphere. He was tall, thin, somewhat tense-looking, and very formal. He immediately lit up a cigarette. I wasn't sure what to make of that. He didn't ask too many questions, which was a relief. No charade. He had my "history" from Dr. Hoffman. He knew why I'd been referred to him. Diagnosis: lupus with fulminating thrombocytopenia; suggested therapy: splenectomy. Dr. Hoffman had probably also told Dr. Cheever something about me as a person. Otherwise he might not have been quite so direct.

After explaining the procedure he announced, plain as day, "I can't give you any odds . . . one way or the other."

It was hardly encouraging, under normal circumstances. But I liked Dr. Cheever's no-beating-around-the-bush style. The operation was a last-ditch effort. It was worth trying, but it was not wise to have unrealistic expectations about it. Dr. Cheever's sober prognosis counter-balanced Dr. Ernst's excessive enthusiasm. I knew I was in the right hands.

I wanted to sign myself into Lyman Memorial right then and there. I wanted to get it all over with quickly, regardless of the outcome. Unhappily, the best Dr. Cheever's secretary/nurse could do was to schedule me for May 23, almost three weeks away! It was one thing to agonize for weeks over the decision itself; it was quite another to have to endure, for weeks more, the agony of waiting. My desperation must have been evident. Before I could plead for an earlier date, she said, "We'll let you know if anything opens up before then."

* * *

Tuesday, May 10. "Dr. Cheever's office. Is this Susan? . . . Can you come in for pre-admission testing this afternoon?"

"Sure! Does that mean you were able to reschedule the surgery?" Without time to think about the consequences, I felt elated.

"Yes. You'll have your tests today, be admitted tomorrow, and Dr. Cheever will do the surgery the day after . . . Thursday, the twelfth at 2:30. Just go to the pre-admission testing office any time today. They'll have the forms ready. Good luck."

I was on my way in minutes that seemed more like seconds. Labwork. Paperwork. EKG and chest X-rays. Soon I was back in Thornden.

My father came home early to help me fix dinner, our "last supper" together at home. For a while? Forever? Because of the Medrol, I still couldn't celebrate with alcohol. "Fake" beer had lost its appeal. I settled for a hot fudge sundae, using up the last of the good Swiss chocolate in the most decadent fashion possible.

As soon as the receptionist in Admitting gave me my plastic basket with a cup, tray, and assorted toiletries, I knew that my luck was holding out. The label read "Room No. 5036." One floor down from my last domicile. A private room! It felt almost like home: I knew where the storage spaces were, how the control buttons worked, where the kitchen was across from the nurses' station. It was odd to feel comfortable in a place I once dreaded.

Shortly before dinner, Dr. Cheever came by with his two residents, Dr. Brown and Dr. Kelly. Surgery was scheduled for the next afternoon. In the meantime I would have an IV put in for my steroids, and receive another transfusion of packed red blood cells. None of this was new to me. The gadget I was given for breathing exercises was. I expected something along this line, but I didn't know what. Eva, in her typically pessimistic style, had warned me about the danger of my developing pneumonia after the surgery if I didn't cough regularly and hard. So I was prepared for the respiratory therapist, but not his gift: a plastic cylinder with a ball inside and a tube attached. It looked more like a toy than a life-saving instrument. It *was* a toy!

I spent much of the evening playing with my new contraption, watching the ball go up and down the cylinder, each time trying to push it a little higher. My father took a liking to it, too, taking his turn on the machine during our endless rounds of Scrabble. He had decided to bring the game in tonight. Perhaps he wanted a chance to erase his debts before it was too late.

Alone again after he was thrown out, long after official visiting hours, I wanted to call every friend I had. But I was afraid of becoming too emotional. Instead, I watched the packed red cells dripping into my veins and drifted off to sleep. I woke up around five a.m. and sat up in bed, with difficulty. I wished the surgery had been scheduled for the morning. I felt exceptionally "wired"—no doubt from the intravenous steroids plus the pre-operative adrenaline. I couldn't concentrate on reading. My hands were too shaky for knitting. I didn't want to write any letters, fearing they would sound too morbid. I didn't want Kate, my only friend in town, to cut class for a trip to the hospital. I wondered if I hadn't made a mistake when I gave Yinky strict orders not to come either. Now I wished I wasn't alone.

I was glad to see Dr. Hoffman. There was little shop talk. We just chatted. Dr. Hoffman knew I needed the company, but knew better than to give me a pep talk. As he got up to leave the room, he gave me a loving pat on the top of my head and said he'd come by later. No "Good luck," or "You'll be fine." I appreciated his not behaving unusually on this most unusual day.

I had the rest of the morning to kill. I should have asked for one last session in P.T. with Carol. Instead, I strolled the halls, with my IV pole for support instead of the cane I'd recently become dependent on. A little exercise felt good. But that too made me tired so I returned to my room, and plopped my body into the stiff, but much too deep, armchair at my bedside. A short time later, when I attempted to get up to go to the bathroom, I felt a sharp, shooting, pain in my lower back. I froze, no longer sitting, but not quite standing. Fortunately, a nurse happened to be in the room changing the sheets, ready to help me get back into bed and lie down. Horizontal, the sharp pain became a dull, constant, ache; the slightest movement bringing on another piercing twinge.

I couldn't have picked a worse time for this to happen. Already the subject of many a "she-doesn't-look-so-sick" stare from the nurses, I now encountered still more disbelief. This "spasm," they implied, was in my head, not in my back. It was nothing more than fear of the surgery. When Dr. Brown and Dr. Kelly arrived on their morning rounds they found me in bed, in agony. They seemed to believe my pain was genuine, but they were unwilling to give me anything for it, already uneasy about my tolerance for general anesthesia and not wanting to aggravate the possibility of complications. Their explanation didn't make my back feel any better, but their understanding made me less angry.

My father arrived around noon, planning to spend lunchtime playing one last game of Scrabble. He hadn't done as well the previous night as he had hoped. But I couldn't sit up. He insisted we play anyway. Winning another ten dollars, at this moment, wasn't what I needed.

He accompanied me to the pre-op waiting area, allowed there more for being a physician than a father. He leaned over the stretcher and kissed me. How I wanted to hug him in return.

* * *

Twenty-four hours later I was awake, and evidently alive. I had survived the splenectomy.

Dr. Cheever came by with his residents to inspect his work. Everyone, myself included, was surprised, and, at least for the time being, pleased. The long-term outcome, of course, remained uncertain, but I came through the operation remarkably well. My first post-splenectomy platelet count was 100,000. Fantastic! That afternoon, just one day after the operation, I was walking, holding onto my IV pole on one side and a nurse on the other. As the weekend progressed, so did I.

"Are you feeling as good as your numbers look?" Dr. Cheever inquired as he greeted me on his rounds early Monday morning.

"That all depends on how good *they* look!" I was feeling pretty chipper. I wasn't sure how much of this was genuine and how much artificial. Now I was getting not only steroids but also morphine! My next platelet count was 289,000. A miracle! I probably hadn't had that many platelets since being diagnosed with lupus in 1969. Dr. Ernst sure knew what he was talking about, at least as far as thrombocytopenia was concerned.

"Unless Dr. Hoffman thinks otherwise, you can go home tomorrow," Dr. Cheever said.

I could scarcely believe my ears.

When Dr. Hoffman arrived in the evening, he had already spoken to Dr. Cheever about my incredible progress. Now he could see for himself.

"Home *tomorrow*," I beamed. "Can you believe it?"

"So, when are you going to start thinking about becoming a contributing member of society again . . . and go back to work?" I could tell Dr. Hoffman wasn't joking.

"I think I'll need to get rid of *that* first, no?" I said, pointing to my cane. Not wanting to dampen his enthusiasm—or my own—I said nothing else. I knew I still had a long road ahead of me. I didn't know how long.

Fourteen

> Home is the only place where you can go out and in. There are places you can go into, and places you can go out of, but the one place, if you do but find it, where you may go out and in both, is home.
> —George MacDonald

Once I was at my father's house again, I was convinced—for the first time since this episode began in January—that I was recovering. I looked forward to the summer ahead as a good time for recuperating. After less than a week out of the hospital, I called Judith, my supervisor at the library, and told her I'd be back at work for the beginning of the fall semester. Frank, Linda, and Kelly came up to see the improvement with their own eyes, and report back that I wasn't kidding. And when Kate came over a few days later and helped my father cook dinner, she joked, "Isn't this more fun than planning a funeral!" My first weekend out of the hospital seemed too good to be true.

My father and I went out for what started as a simple Sunday drive but turned into a little shopping trip. He liked me to help him pick out his clothes and wanted to go to his favorite discount clothing store. He really didn't need me. He always came home with either a grey suit or a navy-blue blazer. Soon it would be summer, which narrowed it down to the navy-blue blazer category. I could never understand why he liked to shop at this warehouse. He could well afford to shop in a real men's store, and often did. But I think he also enjoys the idea of a $99 suit on a famous man.

As we stepped inside the cavernous store, I saw the stairs. There couldn't have been more than ten—with a big, heavy, metal banister running down the middle.

"I'm not sure this is such a great idea," I mumbled, staring at the steps. My father was already at the top, giving me an encouraging, "You can do it" look. Cane at one side, railing at the other, I ascended, one step at a time. It was just like at home. I no longer felt exhausted by a flight of stairs, as I did when I was so anemic. But replacing my muscle strength was going to take considerably longer than replacing my red cells. As I got to the last step at the top, I felt an intense pain in my lower back, which quickly turned into a dull, constant ache. It felt just like what had happened at the hospital. What *was* this?

"I think I pulled something in my back on the way up these damned stairs," I announced. I wouldn't have been able to hide it anyway.

Looking a bit guilty, my father could only admit, "Maybe this *was* too much activity so soon?"

Maybe. More likely, it made no difference. I was an accident waiting to happen.

Back at home, I immediately took a Darvon. Dr. Cheever had prescribed this for post-operative pain—abdominal, he thought. I tried to lie down and rest, but couldn't get comfortable. I tried some of my physical therapy exercises, but they seemed to aggravate the pain. I noticed I felt better standing. But I had to sit down, sooner or later. When I did, on the toilet, I could hardly get up again. Time for another Darvon.

A glass of Scotch might have helped more, but I was still on too high a dose of Medrol for that. Soon the pain in my back became nearly unbearable, no matter what I did. I didn't have to complain. My father could always tell how I was feeling, even when I said nothing.

"I think I should call Hoff," my father announced after dinner, his fingers already dialing the phone.

I really didn't like it when he interfered this way, calling him at home when there was no emergency. Maybe as one doctor to another this was acceptable behavior. But why call Dr. Hoffman *now*? What did he expect him to do?

"I think that's pointless . . . Why not wait until the morning?" But he had already finished dialing.

After barely saying hello, my father handed *me* the phone. "*I* wanted to wait until tomorrow morning to call you," I hastened to say. "I think I did something to my back . . . strained something? Just going up some stairs." I didn't dare say *outside* the house. "I've taken a couple Darvon. They don't help much."

"You probably pulled a muscle," Dr. Hoffman responded, calmly. "If you have any Valium at home, take one before you go to sleep . . . and call me in the morning."

When I awoke Monday morning, I couldn't get out of bed. Not even to go to the bathroom.

"DADDY!" I yelled as loud as I could so as to carry through the closed doors of each of our bedrooms. He stumbled, half asleep, into my room. He must have taken a Valium too, to calm his nervousness about my back. "Help me get up to go to the BATHROOM!" I begged, hurriedly, about to urinate all over the sheets. I wasn't so modest to care if my father saw me on the toilet. Better that than wet, smelly sheets.

Over the years, I had developed the ability to tolerate a lot of pain. Practice makes perfect. As long as I could get around on my own, I had always been willing to endure it. Now I needed help to get up and go to the bathroom. This would pose a problem, and not only for me: I couldn't be home alone this way; but my father couldn't stay home with me either, not twenty-four hours a day, seven days a week. The most immediate, even if not the best, solution would be to bring Yinky over to the house. She could stay with me during the day; my father would be home at night. Of course, at nearly eighty-nine, Yinky wasn't strong enough to help me out of bed. But she could carry a bedpan. I would be *bedridden*. Totally dependent.

As this realization began to sink in, sitting on the toilet waiting for my father to return to help me back to my bedroom, I consoled myself with the rationalization that this was only temporary. It would only last a couple of days. I tried to think positively.

My father went to fetch Yinky, stopping along the way at a drugstore for a bedpan. This must have been the only medical/pharmaceutical item we didn't already own.

Meanwhile, I called Dr. Hoffman to tell him I was no better and didn't think I'd be able to keep my appointment with him the next day.

"Don't worry about that. Stay in bed and rest. I'll come by and see you one day this week on my way home." He sounded too reassuring.

Forty-eight hours later, Yinky was showing Dr. Hoffman the way to my bedroom. The last time Dr. Hoffman and I had seen each other was the night before my discharge after the splenectomy. We were both elated that evening, pleasantly surprised at the apparent success of the operation. It was like sharing the winnings of a lottery. Now someone had broken into the bank and stolen the prize money, without either of us having had a chance to spend a dime!

My bed was strewn with papers, my father's manuscripts he'd given me to edit. My father called this "distraction therapy." Dr. Hoffman gave me a look which said, "That's not what I call *resting*." But he knew I was incapable of being totally idle, even at my sickest.

"I think you should try to stand up. It's been a couple of days."

Before I had a chance to prepare myself for this endeavor, he yanked me out of the bed. Now the pain was excruciating, really unendurable. I was angry. Dr. Hoffman appeared upset, more at the sight of his effort having failed so miserably than at having aggravated my discomfort. I was afraid to say anything, fearing I'd regret it later. At that moment, I wasn't sure I ever wanted to speak to Dr. Hoffman again.

"I'm going to send a lab that makes house calls here tomorrow. We need to keep an eye on your numbers and start thinking about cutting down the Medrol again."

My back was hurting. I was mad. But I realized that, right now, cutting down the steroids was the most important issue.

* * *

I wished Eva and Michael had picked a better time for a visit. But they had very busy schedules and had planned a long Memorial Day weekend in Thornden months before. Only a week earlier we had all looked forward to celebrating my recovery, perhaps even bending the rules and going out to dinner at a posh restaurant. Instead, Eva, Michael, Yinky, and my father took turns delivering food to me upstairs, where I remained confined to bed. At least now I could sit up at the edge of the bed, and take a few steps with the walker that once belonged to Yinky. She had used it temporarily, years before when her arthritis-plus-osteoporosis had flared up. I didn't like the idea of borrowing my grandmother's walker any more than she liked the idea of lending it to me. Clearly, this was no solution. We needed to hire outside help, not only to be at home with me during the day, but also to allow everyone else the freedom to get away. Enter home aides.

If this solution was the best available, it was not by much. But it was easy to arrange. All my father had to do was call one of the many companies listed in the Yellow Pages under "Nurses." All the companies offered nurses for standard eight-hour shifts—seven to three, three to eleven, eleven to seven; they could provide aides, licensed practical nurses (LPNs), or registered nurses (RNs); my insurance would cover 80 percent of the cost if I hired an LPN or RN. Money was the least of our concerns. My father would have been happy to pay for some assistance. Still, I had learned how to make the most of my insurance "benefits."

From my father's perspective, the arrangement didn't look so bad. From mine, it was another story. By now I was so disagreeable that everyone and everything made me mad. I found these series of strangers coming in and out of the house exceedingly offensive. Bad enough that they were in the house. Why did they have to spend so much time in *my* room? I suppose they were only trying to earn their wages by doing something for me. But I found myself, in my own home, in my own room, a prisoner, stripped of all my privacy. Just because I needed someone to bathe me in bed and shove a pan under me didn't mean I needed the constant companionship of a complete stranger. There had to be a better way to deal with this problem.

We had to find a more stable, at least semi-permanent arrangement to help me cope with day-to-day living. My father agreed. Regardless of what Dr. Hoffman was saying—and he wasn't saying much, other than "It's probably just a muscle spasm"—my virtually total incapacity had already gone on too long to be considered temporary. An entire week had passed with me flat on my back, in utter agony most of the time, dependent on my father and grandmother, and so-called nurses' aides. Actually, my father was getting up in the middle of the night to bring me a bedpan whenever I yelled for help! We had been through a great deal together. He had always given much more than any father—any person—might be expected to give. But this was the limit—for both of us. As we had so many times before, my father and I had to figure out some other solution, together. Each of us had to give—give up—something.

We decided that I would return to Yinky's house and he would try to hire someone on a regular basis to help out during the day. Much as I dreaded going back to stay at my grandmother's, I knew I had to accept this compromise for my father's sake. He could not continue to chauffeur Yinky to his house, arrange for a temporary home aide every day, play nursemaid at night, and do his own work. It was bad enough I couldn't escape the patient role. There was no need for him to become a full-time caretaker.

My father set out to find this miracle worker we were looking for. He was resourceful, as always, and very lucky. He knew someone, who knew someone, who knew someone. At the end of this daisy-chain—after just one day of persistent inquiries—he came home from the office with the news that one of his colleagues knew a young woman finishing nursing school, who was looking for a temporary job. He had already made an appointment for her to come to the house.

Dorothy came the next day for an interview. At first I was surprised that my father had arranged such a meeting. I was so happy with the news that I assumed he had *hired* someone. I realized, however, that this formality was appropriate. We were contemplating hiring someone to spend the better part of every day with me—and with my grandmother—helping both of us, and indirectly, my father as well. And, of course, she too deserved the opportunity to "interview" us. After all, what we needed and wanted was not exactly a job requiring a nurse's training. In truth, we were looking for a glorified babysitter for a twenty-seven-year-old woman!

Dorothy was in her late thirties, tall, attractive, with long, wavy hair, and a soothing voice. She was large enough, especially by my standards, to be well able to help me physically. At the same time, there was something amazingly gentle and comforting about her demeanor. She was curious about my lupus, my present condition, my prognosis, and the physical therapy I might need. And she was genuinely attentive to what *we* wanted. She was too good to be true. My luck hadn't been going so well lately.

Dorothy proved to be a turning point. We all—my father, Yinky, and I—took an instant liking to her; and she to us, we felt. Amidst our friendly conversation, it was almost awkward to bring up the issue of money. Based on my experiences with private duty nurses in the hospital and home aides, I had a rough idea of what to offer. The range was between seven and ten dollars an hour. At this point, Dorothy wasn't even a licensed practical nurse. She agreed to work for $6.50 an hour and was willing to come from nine to five, Monday through Friday. Although Dorothy would receive less than any "professional" I could have hired, she cost me more. My major medical insurance would pay for 80 percent of the cost for home care, but only if I hired a *real* nurse. It was a choice I had to make. Thankfully, I could afford to have the choice. Still, it was ironic that only by wasting money for a type of service I didn't need could I have saved money. However, while I might have saved money by buying a higher level of service than I actually needed, I would have received a lower level of service in terms of what I really wanted. If ever there was a time to live by the principle, "You pay for what you value and value what you pay for," this was it.

* * *

Eva and Michael spent the last day of their vacation helping move me to Yinky's. Along the way, we took care of a few medical appointments. Eva helped me get dressed. Michael carried me like a sack of potatoes down the stairs to the car. It was a good thing the doctors' office building adjoining Lyman Memorial supplied complimentary wheelchairs for our rounds: to the lab, to Dr. Cheever for a post-operative appointment; to Dr. Hoffman for a routine check-up; and to an examination by an orthopedic surgeon.

I was—we all were—anxious to find out what was really wrong with my back. My father had wanted me to see Dr. Nichols, a professor of orthopedic surgery at Mansfield General he knew well. I recalled seeing him once, years earlier, for a sprained ankle; my grandmother saw him more frequently for her arthritis and osteoporosis. Unfortunately, Dr. Nichols was out of town, as he often was. So my father called Dr. Farrell, another colleague at Mansfield General. It didn't make any difference to me. Whoever I saw would order X-rays of my spine to determine what was wrong. This did not require any special expertise. My indifference probably came across to Dr. Farrell in an unflattering way. He must have also known that he was only being consulted as a second choice. It was not the prescription for a particularly pleasant visit.

Eva wheeled me to the X-ray department, cleverly exchanged my dress for a hospital gown while I remained seated, and held onto my good-luck onyx necklace I should have left at home. The technician took over and wheeled me towards the X-ray table. I gazed at it, and then up at him.

"Okay," he began, "we're going to take some films of your spine.

Can you hop up on the table for me now?" If this was supposed to be a joke, it wasn't very funny.

Drugged and in pain, I wasn't in the mood. "Look," I said, nastily, "if I could do *that*, would I be *here*?"

The X-rays showed I had suffered two compression fractures in the lower back, the lumbar portion of the spine, at L-3 and L-4—the vertebrae relied upon most for supporting the back. These fractures together with my weakened abdominal and leg muscles made it virtually impossible for me to walk.

So, this time Dr. Hoffman had been wrong. My agonizing back pain was not due to a muscle spasm. I had a "broken back"! We both knew, without either of us saying a word, why this had happened. My bones had become brittle from the months of megadose Medrol—on top of fourteen years on lower-dose, but uninterrupted, steroid therapy. The vertebrae had *collapsed spontaneously*. That they might continue to "rearrange" by smaller collapses was also possible, indeed probable—regardless of what I did. The vitamin D and calcium supplements I'd been taking in recent months were a good idea, but they were too little, too late.

In any case, I had to regain my muscle strength and reduce the steroid dosage. These two goals were mutually reinforcing. The less steroids I ingested, the more my muscle strength would return, spontaneously. Physical therapy could greatly hasten this process, of course. But with acute compression fractures of my spine, I couldn't do any exercises. It was a dilemma. Since the splenectomy, I had managed to go from 80 milligrams of Medrol a day to 64—an appropriate reduction over a two week period of time.

I was afraid when Dr. Hoffman proposed another cut, to 40 milligrams a day, so soon. I had experienced the "flying" feeling from high dose steroids many times. It was irritating, but at least it could also be exhilarating. I'd never come down from so steep a high before. I didn't know what it meant to crash.

Fifteen

Remember that pain has this most excellent quality: if prolonged it cannot be severe, and if severe it cannot be prolonged.
—Seneca

The next weeks and months seemed filled with just three things: agonizing pain from the compression fractures of my spine, overwhelming depression from steroid withdrawal, and a fuzzy head and queasy stomach from codeine and Valium—to make this hell survivable. As I look back, I can recall exactly what was going through my mind, how I felt with every simple movement, like turning from side to side in bed, or just trying to lift my head up from the pillow. I still cannot understand how I endured it. This was worse than the ordeal I had gone through from January to May. Before the splenectomy, I was in no real pain, was reasonably independent, and at the worst moments could take solace in the thought that I was going to die. It would be the end of my suffering. That was comforting.

Although I was beginning again to doubt that I would fully recover, I knew I was *not* going to die—not from osteoporosis and a cracked spine. But I was in constant pain and utterly dependent on others for the simplest human needs. Now I *wanted* to die, more than at any time in the months before, when death had just been something likely to *happen* to me. There was only one person who knew that this was how I felt: my father. Our discussions on the subject were almost as agonizing and unrelenting as the pain in my back—for my father probably more than for me. My relentlessly repeated assertions that I wanted to kill myself— and my pleadings for his assistance—bore no resemblance to the dignified, intellectual conversations on the right to suicide that had kept many a dinner party at our house going into the wee hours in years past.

The irony was that killing myself months ago, when I was terminally ill, would have been "acceptable." While I believed in the libertarian philosophy of suicide, I recognized that in our society only the terminally ill have a "right" to suicide. For the healthy, it is still a stigma.

As June dragged on, I seemed to be getting worse by the day. The thought of killing myself became an obsession. I should have killed myself when I was physically able to do it. Now I *couldn't*, not by myself. I kept badgering my father with, "I've had enough. I want out, *now!*" One night, his patience exhausted, our colloquy came to a head.

"You don't expect *me* to help you to kill yourself, do you?" he said, half in frustration, half trying to show me the absurdity of my request.

"I can't do it alone," was all I could say.

"Well, you should have thought of that *before*. You know you can always do it *later*. Your muscle strength *will* return. You can *always* kill yourself, you know that."

* * *

Dorothy arrived at Yinky's each morning around nine. Half-awake in one of the back bedrooms, I could pretend to not overhear their daily conversation about me. Dorothy did as much good for Yinky as she did for me. In addition to providing a sympathetic ear, she also gave my grandmother a chance to get out of the house during the day and go about her own routine, which my presence had once again disrupted.

Despite my pain, I couldn't remain on my back twenty-four hours a day for much longer. Inactivity would only aggravate the steroid myopathy. It was time to get fitted for a brace that would support my lower back and facilitate my mobility. Dorothy found a medical supply store that would send someone to the house. She showed the man from Harry's Pharmacy into my room and together they helped fit me into the brace. Actually, they fit the brace *onto* me. It was a scene from *Gone with the Wind,* except instead of Scarlett it was me who was being laced by Mammy into an intricate yet primitive-looking corset that must have weighed a couple of pounds. It was as long as my entire torso, with tiny hooks-and-eyes all the way up the front, from my sternum down to my pelvis; criss-crossed shoelace-like patterns on each side, which pulled at the hips to tighten; a pair of one-inch steel metal bands down the back, reaching from just below my shoulders to just above my buttocks. Dorothy laid the corset on the bed and I rolled onto it; she fastened the front, tightened the sides, and turned me over on my stomach so the metal "stays" could be shaped to match the curve of my spine. I felt the corset stabilizing my back instantly. It supported my entire body. But with my abdominal muscles soft as butter, I was even less able to sit up on my own with the corset on than without it.

I had never been so dependent on a prosthesis so big, so cumbersome. Having to walk with a cane was nothing by comparison. The cane was an external support. The corset was like a part of my own body. I now realized, more clearly than I ever had, how my father must feel with his false teeth or my grandmother with her hearing aids. Every such prosthesis, each in its own way, is profoundly annoying to wear. Each gives the wearer the sense of a foreign part being attached to his body. And yet each is essential for enhancing or facilitating a basic bodily function.

Dr. Hoffman was satisfied when the latest results from the lab indicated my lupus was under control. "I think we should reduce the Medrol again, down to 32 milligrams a day," he said when I called to check in, only one week after the last reduction.

I didn't know whether to look forward to feeling stronger or to fear being more depressed. So far, each reduction had resulted only in the latter. Physically, I had yet to see any positive effect from the decreased steroid dosage.

"And I want to see you *here* in the office, next week. Ask Jill to make an appointment."

I hadn't even been outdoors since the day Michael carried me into Yinky's house. I didn't see how I'd ever make it all the way to Dr. Hoffman's. Every day for the next week, Dorothy and I practiced. She escorted me out the front door, guided me down three steps, and steered my body about thirty feet while I hung on tightly to the walker. This was not exactly what I would call walking. Once outside, I stood in place for a few seconds, shuffled my feet a few inches, and then stood again while Dorothy lifted the walker for my next step. At this pace, it would take the next week to reach Dr. Hoffman's office!

These efforts aside, I was plainly not getting better, at least not very quickly, not nearly quickly enough to avoid being categorized as suffering from a long-term disability. I had been out of work for four months. I seriously doubted I would be back within the six-month period that constitutes short-term disability. My spirits were not lifted when I received a letter from the University Personnel Office informing me that short-term disability meant temporary disability. The implication was that long-term disability might well be permanent. I was told to file for long-term disability.

So far, while on short-term disability—really "sick leave"—I continued to receive my full salary. This was a benefit I never dreamed any employer offered. I would be paid for six months without working. My health care costs were covered by health and hospital insurance. And I had the security of my father's financial support, if needed. Money was the least of my worries. Nevertheless, I found myself thrust into dealing with a bureaucracy I never imagined having to face, partly because I never envisioned myself so disabled, and partly because I assumed I had all the insurance protection a person in my financial situation would need or could have.

To my surprise, I was a candidate for the federally administered financial assistance program known as Social Security Disability. Indeed, my employer *required* that I apply for Social Security Disability as a part of the university's disability insurance program. I wasted no time calling the local Social Security Administration for the necessary forms and procedures. Instead of being asked anything about my health or disability, I was asked a question I didn't anticipate.

"Miss Szasz, how many quarters have you worked in the last five years?"

I had no idea what "quarters" meant. I said I'd been working since 1976. I saw no point in explaining how much, or how little, I'd actually worked since then.

"That's fine, Miss Szasz. You'll need to come down to our office and fill out the necessary forms."

Come down? I could barely sit up and take a few steps. "I don't think you understood me. I'm applying for *disability* benefits." I raised my voice slightly for effect. "I'm *completely* disabled. Can't you *mail* me the forms?"

"I'm sorry, Miss Szasz, but you'll *have* to come in and fill out the forms in person."

I couldn't believe my ears. I was *disabled* enough to be eligible for benefits, but was supposed to be *able* to go to a downtown office building and appear in person to fill out a bunch of forms. If I were that mobile, how could I be considered *disabled*? Perhaps this was part of a deliberate weeding out process, designed to protect the system against malingerers. I persisted. Eventually, I found someone at the other end of the line who was willing to mail me the forms.

* * *

Nearly everyone is familiar with Social Security—especially at election time when politicians argue about it—but most people think of it solely as a retirement benefit. People expect to retire and usually plan for it. Disability is not something healthy people like to contemplate. No doubt many people fear it even more than death. Even I, who had already spent more than one-half of my life "sick" and prided myself on being informed and responsible about my illness, knew shamefully little about what might happen to me if I became disabled.

As my initial phone call to the Social Security Administration illustrated, the SSA—the very source of the necessary information—proved to be unreliable. The situation I encountered reminds me of the reports on the accuracy of the information provided by the Internal Revenue Service's 800 telephone number. Studies have shown that they give incorrect answers to queries as much as 40 percent of the time. There are similar studies, with similar results, about the answers given at library reference desks. Not where *I* work, of course!

The personnel officer at the library, lacking experience with disability claimants, was equally unhelpful. My physicians (like, I suspect most others) were completely unfamiliar with these non-medical aspects of medical disability. Once again, the burden of gathering and digesting the relevant information fell on the patient. I made more telephone calls to the Social Security Administration, wrote to their offices for all the material they could send, and talked my colleagues at the library into doing some legwork for me. In this way, I learned not only about disability insurance, but also about the operations of one of the government's largest bureaucracies.

The federal government administers two types of income maintenance programs potentially available to those with chronic illnesses: Social Security Disability (SSD), and Supplemental Security Income

(SSI). They differ mainly in their eligibility requirements. SSD is available only to those with an adequate record of employment, regardless of financial need; SSI is available only to those who do not meet the work history requirements of SSD and whose incomes are low enough to qualify for financial assistance. Although I didn't understand it at the time, this was the reason why the first question I was asked over the telephone concerned my record of employment, not the state of my ill health. I should have been asked another question at the same time: my age. Even the federal government is not so mindless as to expect a twenty-seven-year-old (as I was at the time) to have worked as many "quarters" as a person ten or twenty years older. For each year under the age of thirty-one, the work-time required to qualify is prorated. I had enough Social Security "credits" for someone my age.

As I studied the pertinent pamphlets from the Social Security Administration and other sources, I learned that nine out of ten workers in the United States are covered by SSA's disability program, and that nearly two-thirds of all disability claims are denied on the first application! Many others fail to collect benefits because they are misinformed, cannot negotiate the complex application process, lack the necessary information, and give up in frustration.

I had to file my disability claim as soon as there was reason to believe I might not be back at the library within a year from the last day I had worked. A shorter period of disability, regardless of severity, was not covered by SSA. Completing the application forms is no easier than obtaining them. An example may be helpful here. The following question appears on the first page of the application: "What is your disabling condition?" What is one supposed to answer here? I could have simply put down "systemic lupus erythematosus." But that would not have identified the precise nature of my present disability. After all, I'd had lupus for fourteen years. It alone didn't make me disabled. However, in the last few months I had suffered from an unrelenting and severe fever of unknown origin, life-threatening thrombocytopenia, the consequences of splenectomy, and the disastrous result of massive steroid therapy. I had severe steroid myopathy, pronounced osteoporosis, and multiple compression fractures of the spine. This package of conditions constituted my present disability.

The point is that the so-called side effects of a treatment—a euphemism for undesirable effects—may be no less important causes of disability than the illness itself. I listed all the medications I was taking, the total number so large I needed to attach a separate sheet of paper. Other relevant items that support a disability claim and may be overlooked include the use of a cane or a walker, a brace for back support, a TENS (transcutaneous electric nerve stimulator—more on this presently) for pain relief, and prescribed physical therapy.

I found myself really getting into the gory description of every little detail. While the questions were directed towards my present disability, I saw no reason to ignore the chronic nature of the illness that led up to it. To be sure, this was my first lupus flare severe enough to warrant a disability claim. Still, my medical history, covering more than a decade, was essential for the documentation. I listed the initial date of diagnosis fourteen years ago, the wide range of potentially toxic drugs I had been treated with, and my two prior hospitalizations.

Even with nothing to do all day, it took me nearly a month to complete all the Social Security forms. It was one of the few useful tasks I had accomplished since landing on my back.

* * *

All the while, my sense of well-being continued to deteriorate. The rapid steroid withdrawal combined with the constant ingestion of narcotics had a ruinous effect on both my body and mind. Objectively, I was improving: My lab findings were less alarming, I was past the time for post-operative complications, and my lupus was under firm control again. But I felt destroyed, physically and mentally.

During the whole month of June I walked no more than a few yards in my grandmother's driveway. More often, I could go no further than the foot of the steps of the front door. Once, I went to Dr. Hoffman's office, assisted by Dorothy and a wheelchair ambulance service ironically called ABLE. It was a good thing she was there to supervise the van's driver, who was ready to toss me into the car the way airline baggage handlers throw suitcases onto the tarmac.

Dr. Hoffman told me, as he always did, how good I looked. This time he also praised the few slow steps I took across the examining room, and tried to cheer me up with a glowing report from the lab. But I was not in the mood. Dr. Hoffman had decided to reduce my steroids to 24 milligrams of Medrol a day for one week, and 20 thereafter. He also suggested I wear the brace a little less each day so as not to rely on it too much. The announcements fell on deaf ears. I hated the contraption but had quickly grown dependent on it. Now *that* wasn't good for me. And as much as I wanted, intellectually, to continue decreasing the steroids for the sake of my body, I dreaded its consequences on my mind. How much "lower" could I go? How much more depressed could I feel? My body had suffered miserably from the effects of taking the steroids; now my mind was suffering miserably from the effects of not taking them. I think I stopped listening to Dr. Hoffman. Instead, my mind wandered to my father's most vivid word of wisdom: "Later."

Dorothy was much more cheered by Dr. Hoffman's report than I. She wanted to take me out to lunch to celebrate. I didn't have the heart to refuse. Besides, she was steering the wheelchair. The doctors' office building wasn't far from some of the campus hangouts I used to frequent when I was a student at Mansfield University. The weather was pleasant, warm enough for June, and typically grey. I had to admit it felt wonderful to be outside. We found my favorite Middle Eastern restaurant, with easy wheelchair access. It was the first time I'd ever given *that*, rather than the vast choices on the menu, any thought. Once inside I felt comfortable, but disturbed by people turning to stare at the wheelchair. I'd always been fortunate to have an invisible chronic illness. I couldn't say the same for my present disability.

That evening, I relayed all the "good" news of the day to my father. To him, it sounded like progress. He looked happier than I'd seen him look in weeks. I agreed to play just one game of Scrabble after dinner. I lost. It was a bad omen.

* * *

I lasted exactly one month at Yinky's. Physically, I was no better— and no worse. Our best efforts to manage the situation out of the hospital just weren't working. We got through forty hours of Monday to Friday with Dorothy's help. But that left 128 hours of the week without her. I was still unable to get up and go to the bathroom by myself. For a while, I had a private duty nurse at night. But that seemed ridiculous, hiring someone *just* to help me urinate at night, and eventually we agreed we should try to cope without her. That resulted in one of two scenarios. Either I forced myself to not urinate at all during the night, or I yelled for my grandmother to perform her bedpan duties. Until this time, I didn't realize how valuable a skill I'd learned in my one year at MacArthur High School: Fearing for my life in the lavatory, I never went to the bathroom during an entire seven-hour day. The second alternative was to urinate lying on my back, into a bedpan. With my grandmother playing nurse, well, it wasn't very pleasant for either of us. To top it off, Yinky's hearing was pretty well shot, and she refused to wear her hearing aids at night. Even with my voice, which I'm told is remarkably loud for someone so petite, I often couldn't rouse her from her sleep. An ordinary bell would have been useless. My father's ingenuity again came to the rescue. He dismantled a smoke alarm and turned it into a personal wake-up gadget. With a simple touch of a finger, I could make a noise that would wake the dead. There were nights I thought the fire department would arrive before Yinky. I am happy to be a woman. At that time, however, I wished I were a man, so I could have urinated into a bottle without assistance.

I wanted to return to the hospital, not simply because I was unable to go to the bathroom, but because I had reached the point of desperation. I refused to accept the idea that I couldn't get more help in the hospital than at home. Besides, I had given the home-care arrangement the old college try—for a whole month. I was still, functionally, totally dependent. Also, even though I wasn't really "sick," now I wanted the support of being in the patient role. I knew that Dr. Hoffman would not be sympathetic to my being re-admitted to the hospital. As he saw it, I was progressing satisfactorily, however slowly. Being in the hospital, he would argue, is as likely to do one harm as good. It is a good point, as a rule, but it didn't seem true at that moment. I wanted a doctor who would see the situation as I did.

Since my main problem remained intractable back pain and weakness due to steroid-induced osteoporosis and compression fractures of the spine, the logical person to consult was an orthopedic surgeon. Dr. Nichols was back in town. My father called him and he graciously agreed to see me, immediately. It was a Friday morning, the first of July. My father came by Yinky's very early, arriving before Dorothy. By the time she appeared, he had made arrangements for us to meet Dr. Nichols at Mansfield General as soon as we could get there.

My father must have filled in Dr. Nichols on the events of the past month over the phone. I was relieved to be spared having to give a "history." As far as I was concerned, if I had to be physically dependent on others, I might as well reap some benefits from the dependence. Now, I was ready to give in completely. Dr. Nichols—very professional-looking, a few years younger than my father—was extremely polite and reserved. After examining me briefly, he left for a few minutes only to return with a colleague, Dr. Hoskins, a professor of neurosurgery.

Dr. Hoskins was exceptionally kind, poking and prodding me as gently as possible. I didn't understand what he was testing for. He pricked me with a needle in several places and asked if I felt it. He put a tuning fork against my bones and asked if I sensed the vibration. He stroked my skin with cotton. It all seemed incredibly primitive for so sophisticated a specialty. Of course, he was examining me to determine if I had suffered any neurological damage to my spinal cord. He smiled broadly when he finished and announced that there was nothing wrong.

The more rational part of me was immensely relieved. But I was also dismayed. Some diagnosis—any diagnosis—would have lent credibility to my predicament. I must have a *serious* cause for my *serious* pain. I was beginning to wonder if the doctors believed me when I told them how much pain I was in or how poorly I could move. Then Dr. Nichols came back to the examining room. I grit my teeth for some sugar-coated message and the suggestion that I return home to let time take its course. But Dr. Nichols looked me in the eyes and asked, in the most casual tone: "Susan, do you want to stay here, or do you want to be next door?"

In a flash, my mind had gone from no hospital to a choice between two: Dr. Nichols had privileges at both Mansfield General and Lyman Memorial!

"Over *there*, please." I sighed with relief.

* * *

Sunday, July 3, I turned twenty-eight: telephone calls, flowers, birthday balloons. When the nurses realized it was my birthday, they surprised me with a piece of cake that looked too good to have been baked in the hospital's kitchen. Loving gestures, all. But when I discovered the cake came from a party next door, where an elderly woman was "celebrating" her 365th day in the hospital, I nearly choked on it. Was I going to turn twenty-nine in this place?

Early Tuesday morning, an aide from P.T. was at my door to take me to my first session. She transferred me from my bed to a stretcher with the assistance of two "candy-stripers" and we were on our way. As we approached the nurses' station, Dr. Hoffman appeared. It was an extremely awkward moment. Certain that he would be insensitive to my wanting to return to the hospital, my father and I had managed to get me admitted—on Dr. Nichol's "service." I was worried he would be offended by our outmaneuvering him. At the same time, I was pretty fed up, feeling as if he had given up on me. It didn't occur to me until later that he probably felt relieved by this turn of events. He, too, was at his wit's end about what else to do for me. This way I could be someone else's problem for a few weeks.

Dr. Hoffman leaned over the stretcher, put his hand on my shoulder, and didn't say anything—for what seemed like a very long time. He hadn't given up on me! Instead, I sensed his concern that it was *I* who had given up on myself. He was right. I had come very close to crying in front of Dr. Hoffman before, but had always managed to control myself. This time I didn't even try. I broke down and wept. I was relieved, embarrassed, and ashamed. After a few words of encouragement I didn't want to hear, Dr. Hoffman promised he'd come by at the end of the day. I hoped he would.

I collected myself as best I could and tried to prepare myself for physical therapy. The last time I'd seen the P.T. department I had walked through the doors on my own two feet, aided only by a cane. Now, I came by stretcher. Some improvement. The operation (splenectomy) was a success, but the patient's musculoskeletal system died!

I was one of the first patients that morning. Carol, the therapist I'd spent so much time with earlier in the spring, saw my name on the patient list before spotting me over in a corner.

"SUSAN . . . what's *happened* to my favorite noodle?!"

"Well, Carol," I said, "I guess you could say the noodle dried out and cracked."

Carol understood my present predicament without my having to say another word. Did her somber face mean that she, too, thought I might not recover? I found some comfort in what I took to be her recognition and acceptance of my situation. Here was someone who acknowledged that I wasn't okay, even if I wasn't "sick," someone honest enough to tell me I had a lot of work ahead of me.

* * *

During the next five weeks, I spent almost as much time in physical therapy as the therapists. Five days a week, Monday through Friday, I went downstairs each morning after breakfast and returned to my room around noon. Three hours. After lunch, and a brief rest, I returned for two more hours. In the beginning, I didn't get much "therapy," sampling instead every available method of pain relief—hot packs, ultrasound, and transcutaneous electrical stimulation (TENS). I grew particularly fond of the TENS, a bulky and impressive-looking piece of equipment covered with knobs and wires, resembling an elaborate stereo component. Carol would place two large squares of black rubber resembling wet-suit material on my body, one under my abdomen, the other across my back. Wires ran from each square to the "receiver," where the controls regulating the frequency and intensity of the electrical impulses were located. By sending small electrical impulses to a painful area, the nerves are "distracted," reducing the discomfort. The therapists at Lyman Memorial hadn't had many opportunities to use the machine because the instrument was new and many patients didn't like it. I thought it was great.

Soon I got down to serious physical therapy. Carol knew how far to push me, even if I acted too depressed to keep going. She also knew when to stop. We made a good team. I became aware of how differently I was treated from most of the other patients, who were old. However, the difference lay not only in our ages, but also in the philosophy of the doctors who gave the therapists their orders. The old women with compression fractures were in P.T. only to make them more comfortable. "Ambulating" was not a high priority. I was happy that Dr. Nichols, Dr. Hoffman, and Carol took a different approach to me.

By the end of my first week back in the hospital, I wanted to do more, and convinced Carol I was ready to try and stand up. It was a good sign that I felt like testing myself. But it was a bad idea. Carol and another therapist carefully lowered my body off the stretcher, and as soon as the soles of my bare feet hit the tile floor, I screamed so loud we were sure Security would arrive in a second. The pain shot from the tips of my toes straight up to the top of my skull, and down again. I was devastated, and suddenly just as discouraged as I was a week before, maybe more.

I called the library to tell Frank the latest. "My back doesn't seem to be getting better as fast as I'd hoped. I still can't even stand up, never mind walk. You'd better tell Judith I doubt I'll be back this fall." I didn't want to talk to her myself. I might have been overreacting, but I knew I wasn't.

When I returned to P.T. the following Monday morning, Carol had a new piece of equipment for me to try: a "tilt table." She rolled my stretcher up against the table, slid me onto it, fastened the straps at my chest and knees, and turned on the power. Carol could tilt the table at increasingly higher angles, from a flat 180 degrees to an upright 90 degrees. This procedure allowed me to gradually increase the weight on my spine, instead of going from horizontal to vertical in one drastic step.

Carol also gave me a gadget I could take back to my room: a portable TENS unit. The "receiver" fit into the palm of my hand; the rubber-like electrodes measured about one inch by two inches and could be secured on my back with surgical tape. The TENS helped a lot, especially at night. I still took painkillers during the day, but with the TENS I could often sleep through the night without any drugs.

It was a relief to be more in control and less dependent on the nurses, with whom I often had to justify my requests for pain medication because I didn't "look" like I was in so much pain. More important, it was good for me to take as few analgesics as possible. However much they relieved my pain, they also made me nauseous and depressed. With a quiet stomach, the exercise might help bring back my appetite. With a clear head, I might think more about getting better, and less about killing myself.

Exactly twenty-eight days after I checked into Lyman Memorial, Dr. Nichols informed me that my case had been reviewed by the hospital's bed-utilization committee and they had concluded that my condition no longer warranted hospitalization. *They were kicking me out!* I was stunned. I wasn't ready to go home. Not *yet*. Most of the time, the best I could do was sit up all day and, with my brace on and a walker, perhaps get as far as the bathroom, in my own private hospital room. Some days I could walk longer distances in physical therapy, but only accompanied by Carol to "spot" my shaky movements. Despite these improvements, I still couldn't stand long enough to take a shower, still couldn't even put my brace on or get out of bed by myself. Yet my condition didn't justify staying in the hospital. Even so, I had to agree that the committee was right: Although I was disabled, I didn't require *hospital* care.

I broke the news to my father later that morning. He was as alarmed as I, however justified the hospital committee's decision. We had two choices: I could be transferred to a convalescent center, a euphemism for a nursing home; or I could return to Yinky's, again with help from Dorothy. Neither option was very attractive. The former conjured up visions of old people stored away until they die; the latter made me feel I was returning to the misery I had finally managed to escape. Against everyone's advice, I convinced my father to explore the possibility of some other form of "institutionalization." Dr. Hoffman, in particular, strongly opposed this plan. The ambience of a nursing home, however named, he warned, would only add to my depression, which at last was slowly lifting. But the prospect of returning to Yinky's was also unappealing. I believed, falsely as it turned out, that I could receive more intensive physical therapy at a nursing home than I could privately. Finally, there was the financial consideration. It wasn't a question of what we could afford, but of what made more sense. My medical insurance policy specified that if I went to a nursing home *directly* from a hospital, all the expenses would be fully covered. If I left the hospital and was later admitted from home, nothing would be covered.

This time, my father's conscientiousness worked against both our best interests. Had my father dragged his feet a while, investigating the nursing homes in the area, had he not used his professional connections and pulled strings to get me into one of the best when they were all supposedly full—I could have stayed at Lyman Memorial another week or two or three, long enough to be ready to go home. But that was not our style.

In less than a week, my father succeeded in getting me into the Regency—into a *single* room, no less.

But a Hyatt Regency this was not!

Sixteen

> Human felicity is produced not so much by great pieces of good fortune that seldom happen, as by little advantages that occur every day.
> —Benjamin Franklin

On Friday, August 5, I left Lyman Memorial the way I arrived, via the ABLE ambulance service, this time in a wheelchair instead of on a stretcher. It was not much to show for five weeks in the hospital.

The ride from the hospital to the Regency took less than five minutes. A normal person could have walked down the street faster than the ABLE crew moved me. I settled into my private room, Kate at my side for moral support. I didn't think I could face this alone. As she wheeled me down the hall to reconnoiter, we both got a sinking feeling in the pits of our stomachs. There wasn't a person under the age of eighty in sight. Most were sitting idly, staring into space, or moaning. It was not an altogether unfamiliar sight. The halls of Four North at Lyman Memorial, which housed the orthopedic cases, were also strewn with old people, some strapped to wheelchairs, aimlessly sitting out their days. There was one noticeable difference between this nursing home and the hospital: Everyone was dressed in street clothes, a pathetic pretense to treat people as "residents" rather than as "patients."

I thought I would be able to take refuge in my private room. But just like at the hospital, keeping the door to my room closed was a no-no. Every time a staff member came by, he or she would prop the door open and leave it that way. I also thought I'd be able to leave my room when I wanted. There were railings all along the hallways and I decided to try them. Not five feet outside my door, with Kate at my side, we were severely reprimanded. I didn't have "orders" allowing me to do this.

I was glad that Kate stayed through most of my first afternoon at the Regency. It wasn't that I needed her to do anything for me. I needed her as a witness. I doubted anyone would believe my own account of the day's events.

I sat in my wheelchair most of the day, reading, knitting, or "working" on something for my father. When he came around dinnertime, I took one look at the food delivered to my room and suggested we try to walk instead. Maybe the staff would be too busy feeding the more helpless "residents" to notice that one of them was up and about "against orders." Then he went up the street to Burger King for a Whopper, french fries, and a chocolate milkshake. Now I *knew* I was feeling better.

By the end of this boring but strenuous day, I longed for a good night's sleep. This was easier said than done. With my door open, the noises emanating from the other rooms were annoying and unremitting. And the nurses came in to check on me every couple of hours. For what? Wasn't I sent here from the hospital because I wasn't that sick? To top it off, there was a dim light, recessed into the head-board above my bed. I fiddled with every switch I could reach to turn it off. Nothing worked. Of course—it was supposed to stay lit!

For most of the next three days and nights all I could think about was getting out of the place, the sooner the better. I had been so confident I was making the right decision. But I knew I was wrong. I admitted it. As when I had returned home from college, I wasn't about to remain bound by a bad decision, even if it had been my own. I wasn't going to stay in this nursing home for the sole purpose of saving face. When I saw the Regency's medical director Monday morning, I requested that he leave "orders" allowing me to do whatever I wanted in the way of physical activity—including signing myself out when I felt I was ready. He was barely out the door when I asked to be discharged. While I waited for the paperwork to be sorted out and for my father to make the arrangements to pick me up, I went off to physical therapy. After three days cooped up, I needed it.

I returned the same afternoon to Yinky's house—in my father's car. That alone was a significant and reassuring accomplishment. Happily, I went back to "my" bedroom and my father went back to his office. Suddenly all the things that drove me nuts before—the noisy air conditioner switching on and off, the neighbor's dog barking incessantly, Yinky "quietly" putting all the dishes away in the kitchen as soon as I went to take a nap—seemed like minor annoyances compared to the regimen at the Regency. I slept, for the first time in days, like a baby.

I awoke when my father arrived for dinner, struggled to put my back brace on by myself, and made my way to the dining room with my walker—down the long hallway in the middle of Yinky's house, rendered treacherous by a worn oriental runner on the parquet floor. I celebrated with a Scotch, my first in months, although I still wasn't supposed to drink. I felt as if I had escaped from the House of the Dead.

We had a wonderful dinner. I ate the goulash and Sacher torte like a Hungarian refugee freed from a Communist labor camp. I beat my father twice at Scrabble. Then he walked with me back to my bedroom. As I stood by him, he looked happier than he had in a very long time. The last time we'd been in this room together I was lying on my back in agonizing pain, pleading with him to help me kill myself, while he stood there telling me I could always do that "later." I *had* made progress. I was *vertical*, and optimistic about remaining that way. If ever there was a moment for someone to say to me, "I told you so," this was it. I could hear it coming and was ready to say, "You were right." Instead, he said, "You know, I think you've gotten *shorter*."

My father was right again. I had lost 3 inches of my height! More than 5 percent of the total! Down to 55, the same number as the year I was born.

* * *

The first few weeks at Yinky's I still couldn't get up at night to walk to the bathroom. But I could sit up and stand, if I took the time and trouble to put my back brace on. We rented a portable commode from a hospital-supply store, and added that piece of sick-room furniture to my bedroom. I could go to the bathroom on my own again, even if it was an indecorous ordeal. The inelegance of the commode was far outweighed by its usefulness. I was much less dependent and we could dispense with the use of the smoke alarm to wake up Yinky. Dorothy came during the days again, although for increasingly fewer hours each week.

Finally, the reduction in my steroids seemed to be having the effect we hoped for: The worst of my mental anguish was behind me, and

I was slowly getting stronger. I was anxious to hasten my progress. I needed private physical therapy. I called Carol for a referral. It was a wonderful surprise when she offered her own services instead. Maybe she wanted to finish the job she'd started.

Three days a week at five p.m., for an hour each visit, Carol came to Yinky's. My progress during August was dramatic. After the first week I met Carol at the door with my walker. After the second week I waved to her from the dining room picture window, holding up only a cane as I stood on my own two feet. We began spending more time outdoors, first negotiating the front steps of my grandmother's house, then strolling slowly up and down the sidewalk. Carol didn't need fancy equipment to devise innovative forms of exercise. Yinky's house was situated at the bottom of the steepest hill for miles around, and Carol decided I should practice the climb, each day going up a little further.

At the end of August I *walked* into Dr. Hoffman's office, assisted only by Dorothy on one side and a cane on the other. He was speechless.

Having successfully made one trip into town in Dorothy's car, I wanted to get out of the house more. I became adventurous again. Carol agreed that I was ready to return to physical therapy as an outpatient at the hospital. Dorothy could provide the transportation; the outings themselves would be good for me. Soon Dorothy and I started going out to lunch, shopping at the mall, or just going for rides in the car. Once again, I eagerly anticipated the day I could move from my grandmother's house back to my father's. But I wasn't ready yet to handle a whole flight of stairs, up and down, everyday. And a part of me was still afraid of messing up the progress I was making.

* * *

Saturday, September 3, I received a reply from the Social Security Administration about my disability claim: I was scheduled to appear for my physical examination on Tuesday, September 6, at five p.m. I read the letter, took note of the location for the exam, and came to this closing admonition: "Do not bring anyone with you to the examination."

This seemed strange, to say the least. Surely, most people who apply for disability benefits must be *dis-abled*. If this was intended to instill fear of the Social Security system in this applicant, it didn't work.

I had no intention of going to my Social Security examination—or anywhere else—alone.

I called Dorothy. It would have been easier to go with my father. But I wanted to drive home to the Social Security Administration the reality of my disability and dependence. Being accompanied by a nurse seemed more appropriate—and more effective.

Dorothy picked me up, dressed as a professional nurse, in her white uniform. I was dressed as a professional patient, in a corset and with a cane. The only fake touch was that I didn't put on any makeup, something I *never* do. This time I didn't want to look too good. The agenda called for a review of my claim for *disability*, not a demonstration of how well I had adjusted to living with my illness.

As we walked through the dark parking garage, I was glad I hadn't come alone. Even in my healthier days I disliked being in this part of town alone. The Social Security office had a seedy, unkempt air about it. The door was unmarked except for a slightly faded street number. I felt like I was entering an illegal back-alley abortion clinic. Once inside, the atmosphere was equally depressing: a tiny waiting room with barren walls, no windows, more people than chairs.

After a brief wait, the examiner—a young physician, presumably moonlighting for the Social Security Administration—asked me to follow him. He didn't introduce himself. The interrogation that followed was distasteful and demeaning.

"Miss Szasz, how did you get here today? Did you drive yourself, ride in a car driven by someone else, or take public transportation alone or with assistance?" The man sounded like a recording.

"I was driven here," I replied, pointing to Dorothy, who had accompanied me into the examining room, without asking permission.

"Are you living alone?"

"I used to . . . until seven months ago." I could have just said "No, I'm living with my father," but I wanted to emphasize that my living arrangements had changed because of my present condition.

"What household chores do you perform, if any?"

I was beginning to wonder when, if ever, we were going to discuss my illness. I knew that, for this review, the nature of my illness was secondary to its disabling effects. I also knew that, in the jargon of the Social Security system, the issue was my ability to engage in "substantial gainful activity," not my ability to resume my job at the library. Did "household chores" constitute "substantial gainful activity"? The question reminded me of something I'd read by Flannery O'Connor:

> You can work, says he [the doctor], but you can't exert yourself. I haven't quite figured this out yet; anyway I am confined to these two rooms and the porch so far and ain't allowed to wash the dishes. I guess that is exerting yourself where writing is officially not.

"I don't help at home with any of that," I responded after a minute's reflection. I considered cooking a hobby, not a chore.

"Let's see how far you can bend over. I'd also like to see you stoop and reach."

I looked at Dorothy and hesitated. I wasn't about to do something here that might cause further injury. "I'm not supposed to bend over," I said as politely as I could. "That's why I'm wearing a corset." I was fully dressed, so the examiner couldn't see this. "And I need the cane for walking. I see a physical therapist, three times a week." I wanted to be sure the examiner knew about these things. The corset, the cane, and the physical therapy were objective, demonstrable, evidence of my disability.

My pain, however, was entirely subjective. Describing pain—especially chronic pain—to another person is difficult if not impossible. It is probably best done by illustrating its consequences: by explaining what you do for it, what it does to you, and what it keeps you from doing.

"What medications are you taking for your pain?"

"Percocet* and Valium."

I knew from my reading that the Social Security Administration puts little faith in the patient's complaint of pain. This is not as unreasonable or inhuman as it may seem. As an ancient Greek philosopher wisely remarked, no one can feel another person's pain. Therefore, no one can ever be certain that a person is, or is not, in pain. A severely injured person may not feel pain, whereas a seemingly uninjured and healthy person may experience excruciating pain. And, of course, a person may *complain* of pain in order to obtain drugs or monetary compensa-

---

*Percocet is a combination of acetaminophen and a narcotic analgesic with properties similar to codeine and morphine. I had switched to percocet because it made me less nauseated than the Tylenol with codeine I took in the hospital.

tion. To resolve the unsolvable problem of verifying or falsifying the claimant's pain, the Social Security Administration has its own standard of proof: Under its guidelines, "prescribed medication for pain is an indicator of the credibility of the client's complaints."*

It is wonderfully ironic that the same federal government that is waging a "War on Drugs" and is calling for a "drug-free America" identifies the use of *prescription drugs* as the single most reliable criterion for verifying an individual's claim concerning pain. Typically, a patient suffering from chronic pain is encouraged by his physician to take as little medication as possible. This is wise. It is better to try to cope with chronic pain by means other than medication. At the same time, medication can be of immense benefit. In our hysterical age concerning drugs, physicians are often reluctant to prescribe pain medication for chronic conditions because of the fear that prolonged use will lead to "abuse" or addiction.

* * *

Two days after demonstrating my disability to the Social Security Administration I set out to demonstrate my increased ability to Dr. Hoffman. This time I wanted to see if I could make it all the way on foot from the parking garage. I knew I still needed some extra feet—Dorothy's two and my third, the cane—but this would be the farthest I'd walked in more than three months. I wanted to do it for myself. And for Dr. Hoffman. As I entered his office, I was greeted by a chorus from the receptionists: "Suzy, you're *walking*!"

Dr. Hoffman looked astonished—at my walking as well as my shrunken shape, but refrained from making any sarcastic comment about my height. Like my father, he loved to tease me, but this was not the time. It was obvious that I had been pushing myself, was getting stronger, and was no longer depressed.

I had hoped all this would get me a nice pat on the back. I expected to hear, "Keep up the good work, and I'll see you in a couple of weeks." But today, Dr. Hoffman's expectations exceeded my own.

---

*Quoted in *A Legal Manual for Lupus Patients*. (St. Louis, MO: Lupus Foundation of America, 1982), p. 28.

"I want you to start driving your car again," he announced, after silently scribbling some notes.

Drive my car? "But I don't think I can open the *door*," I said, bluntly.

Dr. Hoffman looked bewildered: "I don't understand. What do you drive? A truck?"

He wasn't far off the mark. I drove a 1979, *two-door* Chevy Malibu. Buying a two-door car was a seemingly insignificant but, in retrospect, serious mistake—like my father's buying a two-story house. But who goes around thinking about the possibility of being so disabled that he can't climb one short flight of stairs? Or open a car door?

Dr. Hoffman's "order" to drive sounded like enough for one day. But he wasn't finished. "If you're going to return to work in January, you can't just sit around at home for the next three and a half months."

I didn't consider my present routine "sitting around." Ordinary living still seemed like work. I couldn't imagine what Dr. Hoffman had in mind.

"I know the head of the library at the School of Nursing," he continued. "I've already spoken to her about the possibility of your helping out there a few hours a week. I'm going to call her right now and tell her you're ready."

I was dumbfounded, but very pleased. "Sounds interesting. I'm game." What, I wondered, would I *wear*!

"This should keep you out of trouble for a while. I don't need to see you for a month," Dr. Hoffman proposed as I got up to leave. "By the way," he added, "all your lab work looks stable"—it was our favorite expression for an acceptable level of disease activity—"so let's try to get you back on Prednisone again."

I'd been on Medrol since February. Returning to Prednisone now struck me as one more way of putting this episode behind me. Driving again, working again, taking Prednisone again. It all made me feel as though I was getting closer to being back to normal—for me.

* * *

When I arrived at the door of the library at the School of Nursing, I was struck by what a modest operation it was: two small reading rooms with book stacks running along the walls; a small office shared by one librarian and her assistant; a tiny card catalog with a half-dozen drawers. I was used to working in a library system of nearly five million volumes, the reference collection alone totalling more than twenty thousand; a seven-story building the size of a huge department store; seven librarians in my department alone; a card catalog with hundreds of drawers weighing ten pounds each, more than I could safely handle, assuming I could reach them. I wasn't ready for that. But this was the perfect transition. I felt at ease from the very first day. Just getting to the library, "working" for a couple of hours, and getting home again, all on my own, were incredibly satisfying achievements. Being in a library again, around students, answering reference questions—all this helped me remember how my life had been nine months before. The idea of returning to work seemed appealing once again. And possible.

Much as I was scared to admit my progress, perhaps lest I jinx it, my father was even more cautious in his expectations. Illness is frequently a heavier burden on the caregiver than on the patient, a fact often overlooked by patients. In many ways, the events of this year had been harder on my father than on me: the initial crisis, the long uncertainty about whether I would live or die, the dubious therapies, the risky splenectomy, the compression fractures of my spine, and, to top it off, my months of unrelenting depression. It was difficult enough for him to be hopeful when we both thought I was going to die. It was worse still when I wanted to kill myself. However one measures pain, the pain in his soul must have been as great as the pain in my body during those months.

My father had frequent invitations to lecture abroad, all of which he had declined this year. Many months before he had received an invitation to visit Israel in early October. He had never been there. He loved to travel. He also thought it would be a nice gesture to take his mother along. She, too, had been through a lot recently, and she was about to celebrate her eighty-ninth birthday. Yinky was still chipper enough to travel, if accompanied by a more able-bodied person. It would be a wonderful birthday gift. While my father had some doubts about leaving me alone for more than a week, I felt I could manage at his house by myself. It was the next logical step on my road back to living alone, in my own apartment, again.

The last day of September, I drove my father and grandmother to the Mansfield Airport. None of us looked too happy about the impending separation. The walk from the gate back through the terminal to the parking garage was long and lonely. But I could walk, almost normally, except for the cane. I wished I could have gone along. Of course, that option had wisely never been seriously considered. I wondered if I'd made a mistake. Was I really ready to be alone? Or, being alone for the first time in nearly a year, was my anxiety normal?

A part of me had looked forward to these ten days of privacy. But a part of me, evidently, still didn't feel well enough, or confident enough, to enjoy my new-found independence. That was just it: I didn't *feel* independent; I felt isolated. I was still afraid to do many things alone and found myself focusing too much on my lingering pain. I began to wonder if my present level of disability, improved as it was, would remain at this plateau. Would I always feel too frightened to appreciate the joys of privacy and independence I once valued so highly?

Soon my reflections turned morbid. In my mind, I went back to the most agonizing weeks of the year, when I wanted to kill myself but was physically unable to do it. Did I want to end up in that helpless position again? Wasn't *now* the time to act? Wasn't this the "later" that my father had told me would come, when I would have the physical ability to kill myself? I certainly had the time now to think this decision through, carefully.

As many an ancient philosopher has noted, I found the very freedom to commit suicide liberating. The more I thought about how easy it would be to kill myself, the less seriously I considered doing so. I took a short drive to the grocery store and picked out an assortment of exotic junk foods my father disliked. Next stop, the liquor store, for a bottle of good wine. Back at the house, I spread out a decadent feast on the living room coffee-table, arranged the pillows on the sofa so I'd be able to get up without straining, and blared Gordon Lightfoot on the stereo. Eating smoked oysters and sipping Robert Mondavi Reserve Fume Blanc, I thought to myself: So what if you never get any better than this? This life is still worth living!

I wanted to live.

Seventeen

> Experience is not what happens to you; it is what you do with what happens to you.
> —Aldous Huxley

Wednesday, October 5, dawned as a magnificent autumn day. I wanted to see more of the colorful foliage before the weather turned cold and the leaves were off the trees. It was the perfect day to take a drive to Concord. I still didn't feel secure enough to do it alone, or to do it without discussing it with Dr. Hoffman, but he was enthusiastic, and Dorothy was willing to accompany me.

I drove all the way. I pulled into my private parking space, marked with my last name, unoccupied all these months. My apartment looked unchanged, except for the dust. Seeing all my things, exactly as I'd left them, I was glad I'd kept the place all year. At times it seemed like a terrible extravagance, a waste of money to pay rent on an apartment I wasn't using and wasn't sure I ever would again. But had I given up this part of my life, I might have given up entirely on life. I gazed out the window at the valley below. I could see the library in the distance.

Dorothy and I drove around the campus several times before I found a place to park. It was a short but steep walk to the library, and I needed Dorothy at my side more than I had imagined, or liked. I accepted having her with me in medical surroundings—in the hospital, at the Social Security Administration office, seeing Dr. Hoffman. Here, I felt conspicuous with her. I didn't see any familiar faces as I walked, but plenty of eyes were focused on me, and my cane. I thought about the handful of wheelchair-bound students I'd helped in the library and admired their self-confidence and perseverance more than ever.

We stopped outside the front door, so I could catch my breath and collect myself. Someone must have seen us, for I was barely inside, still a good distance from the reference desk, when nearly everyone from the department emerged from the office—and started clapping. The students and faculty looked bewildered. I was overwhelmed.

My visit to Concord was exhilarating. The drive back uneventful. The next day I drove to my temporary "job" at the School of Nursing. I stayed longer than usual and got stuck in rush-hour traffic on the way home to Thornden. Finally at my father's house, I stopped at the top of the driveway to pick up the mail and pulled into the garage. I'd been mulling over what to eat for dinner and realized I probably should have stopped at the grocery store for something more nutritious than smoked oysters. When I stepped out of the car, my appetite vanished. Not two feet in front of me lay a mouse—squashed between the prongs of a trap, face up. It wasn't the first time I'd seen one around the house. Soon after we moved into this suburban home in 1975, some mice got into the house, and left their trappings nearly everywhere, even in the kitchen. That was *it*, for my fastidious father. Never again was a mouse going to get into his house, even if that came with the territory of living in such a beautiful woodsy environment. And he hated cats. So he set out his Maginot Line. That's what he called his strategically arranged traps—in front of the kitchen door, next to the trash cans, by the wood pile. He knew where the mice liked to go from where he'd trapped them before. We never had live mice in the house again. But we had plenty of dead ones in traps.

My first impulse was to call our next-door neighbor, Nina, and ask her to send over her teenage son to do the dirty work. She was very thoughtful, calling me every day, to see if she could do anything for me while my father was away. But this seemed like an unnecessary request. I should be able to transfer a little mouse from the floor into a trash can. No big deal. I looked around the garage for an old glove but instead found another dead mouse!

I knew that my osteoporosis and compression fractures made picking up things from the floor precarious, and that I had to be careful. I had to bend at the knees, not at the waist. Actually, even if I tried, I couldn't move incorrectly: The back brace prevented me from bending at the waist. So the task seemed more distasteful than dangerous. If I could have done it with my eyes closed, I would have. I picked up an old newspaper, approached the first trap, bent down, scooped it up, and threw the whole mess in the trash. Like I'd seen my father do it. I picked up another piece of newspaper, walked to the other side of the garage, bent down, scooped up the trap-plus-dead-mouse and . . . something happened. As I lifted my perfectly aligned body up from its crouched position I felt something snap in my lower back. I didn't just *feel* it; I could *hear* a distinct popping sound. As I straightened up, the pain reverberated through my entire body. It was agonizing. I have no idea where the mouse landed as I flung the newspaper across the garage. I stopped dead in my tracks, numbed by the pain, and too enraged to think clearly. Now what?

There was only one consolation. I knew exactly what had happened. I'd been through this before. I walked gingerly toward the kitchen door. The two steps into the house were sheer torture. I had to get to the telephone, quickly. Since she was right across the street, I called Nina. No answer. I called Dorothy. No answer.

I had promised Dr. Hoffman I wouldn't bother him at home while my father was out of town unless it was absolutely necessary. I dialed his home number. Mrs. Hoffman answered, but I could barely hear her over the commotion audible from the background. How could I be so stupid to call in the middle of dinnertime?

"Hi, I'm really sorry to disturb you at home," I mumbled, before even identifying myself. "It's Suzy . . . Suzy Szasz. Is your husband at home?" My voice was starting to crack, the pain in my back getting the best of me.

"Yes, he's right here. Are you all right?" she asked, realizing I wasn't.

"Not exactly. I think I'd better talk to him." As I heard her yell *"Dick,"* the panic in her voice echoed my own.

"What's wrong?" he asked, too calmly, as he came on the line. Soothing as his voice sounded, I would have felt better had I been able to see his face. I suspected he would underestimate the damage, not from doubting my veracity but in an effort to counteract my own (over)reaction.

"I've compressed a couple more vertebrae. It hurts lower down than the last time. Please, do me a favor, don't say it's 'only a muscle strain.'" I wasn't in the mood to hear *that* again.

"What happened?" he asked, eventually succeeding in interrupting me.

"You're not going to believe this . . . I was picking up a dead mouse in the garage, and as I stood up, my back just 'snapped.' Honest."

After a long silence on the other end of the line, while Dr. Hoffman no doubt was restraining himself from laughing, he inquired, jokingly, "You couldn't find a broom?" Realizing why I had called just *then*, he became more serious, and more practical: "You're alone, aren't you?"

"Yes. But I'm trying to get someone to come over for the night. So far I haven't succeeded. I *know* I won't be able to stand up in the morning."

"Do you have any Valium left?" he asked, assuming I still had some. "Take one, get yourself into bed, and lie down."

"But I don't want to take any Valium. It will only make me depressed." I probably would have disagreed with anything he'd said. I knew perfectly well that the five milligrams of Valium was meant to make the muscles in my back relax. I was just too upset.

Dr. Hoffman was in good form: "You're *already* depressed. Take the Valium for your *back*! I'll call you later tonight to make sure you're all right. Okay?"

I hung up and dialed Dorothy again, still standing by the kitchen phone, shifting my weight slightly from foot to foot so as to alleviate the stiffening in my spine. Keep standing, I said to myself, or you'll never make it up the stairs.

"Thank God you're there. I picked up a dead mouse and cracked my back again. I can barely move. Can you come over *as soon as possible* and spend the night?"

Somehow I made it upstairs, wisely stopping in the bathroom along the way, and got myself into bed—slowly. It was a torturous effort. I knew the next time I had to "go," it would be in a bedpan. I was reminded of a story Dr. Hoffman had told me when I first hurt my back in May. He too had had his share of back problems, from a disc, and one time was forced to crawl out of his car, into his house, and up a flight of stairs on his hands and knees. Thankfully, I had everything I needed within an arm's reach from my bed: telephone, television remote control, water, Valium. I turned on the TV and swallowed one 5-milligram tablet, sipping as little water as possible so I wouldn't need to go the bathroom too soon.

Before I knew it, Dorothy arrived. Fortunately, she had a key to the house. She found me upstairs in bed, semi-drugged. I didn't want to talk much. Dorothy let me know I could just holler when I needed her. I managed to sleep through the night, no doubt in part to avoid waking Dorothy for the sole purpose of bringing me the bedpan. The Valium helped. Still, I expected to wake up from the need to urinate, not from the bed vibrating. The whole house was shaking.

There was a large quarry only a few miles from the house. Maybe they were blasting. I turned my head to look at the clock: 6:30 a.m., too early for blasting. I picked up the TV remote control and tuned in on an early morning news program: "The area around Mansfield was just affected by the shocks of a small earthquake, centered several hundred miles from here. The first in decades. . . ." At least I wasn't going crazy.

Although my lower back felt tight as a knot, everything else, above and below, felt all right. I could roll from side to side, move my legs off the edge of the bed, push my torso upright with my arms, and sit up. A complicated but remarkably effective technique Carol had taught me. My bones were as brittle as ever, but at least my muscles were stronger. As long as I kept both hands at my side, on the bed, I could minimize the pain by relieving the pressure on my spinal column. Standing was another matter. Walking to the bathroom, even with help, was clearly out of the question. I resigned myself to sinking, once again, below the "bottom line" of independence.

By three p.m. I was back in Lyman Memorial. I had anticipated some negotiating with Dr. Hoffman over the necessity of my being hospitalized, but this time he didn't disagree. I had just enough time to call the hospital television service and have my room connected. God forbid I'd have to miss "Dallas," not to mention an entire weekend without the news. At least by now I knew the ropes. I also knew how to pull a few strings. I called Carol in P.T. and had her put me on the schedule for Monday morning—without waiting for Dr. Hoffman to write the orders!

"Carol? You're not going to believe this, but I'm *upstairs*." By now she knew me well enough to recognize my voice.

"*Susan? Now* what did you do?!" Carol is my only friend who never calls me "Suzy."

"Get up here when you're finished for the day and I'll tell you the whole story. But you have to promise not to laugh—or to make me laugh. It *hurts* when I laugh."

When Dr. Hoffman arrived shortly after five, Carol was visiting, the two of us chatting and eating the last of the hazelnut torte I'd brought back from the best bakery in Concord. He was clearly unhappy that we hadn't left him a piece.

"You were right," he announced, having just read the X-ray report, "Compressed vertebrae. It looks like you've taken care of everything else without me."

I suppose I had. But as soon as Carol left and Dr. Hoffman and I were alone, my cheerful facade began to crumble.

"I guess I've really messed things up. Everything was going so well. I even made it to my apartment and the library the other day." I realized I hadn't had a chance to tell him any of my good news before hitting him with the bad. "Now it will probably take me another month to get back on my feet again . . . almost Thanksgiving . . . I'll never make it back to work by the beginning of January!"

Sensing my despair, Dr. Hoffman tried to comfort me with some words of wisdom. "It's not going to be like the last time. You've been through it, so you *know* you will walk. And your muscles are a lot stronger now than they were after the splenectomy. You'll still be back at work in January. And you'll be out of here in a week, tops."

I was skeptical. But he was right. This time I was more angry than depressed. I was angry that I had interrupted my progress, not despondent that I was making none. Still, a week seemed such a short period that I wondered if he was humoring me, giving me false hopes so I *wouldn't* get more depressed.

"Have you called your father yet to tell him the news?"

Dr. Hoffman must have been the nth person to ask me that question, to all of whom I had firmly replied, "No! I don't plan to. And don't *you* dare."

At no time did I consider telephoning my father in Israel. The news could only upset and worry him. And how! Why should I do that? It was already Friday evening here, almost Saturday morning in Israel. My father was scheduled to leave there early Monday morning. If I called now, he would end up spending his last twenty-four hours abroad trying, probably unsuccessfully, to return *one* day earlier than planned. There was no point in that.

Our plan was that I would pick up my father and grandmother at the airport on Monday evening. He would call from JFK as soon as he landed, as he always did. He would be beside himself when he didn't find me at home. The important thing was to make sure that anyone my father called next would know my whereabouts. That meant I had to call Eva, which I was planning to do in any case, after dinner. No point in alarming her, either. She was in the middle of the day at work.

* * *

My back was to the door and my eyes were glued to the "Today Show" Monday morning, so I didn't notice Dr. Hoffman until he was right in front of me, staring down at my breakfast tray.

"How did you get a bagel and cream cheese?" he asked, baffled.

By round four, I'd learned quite a few things about how to make life more tolerable in the hospital, among them how to order food that wasn't on the menu. As long as they had it in the cafeteria downstairs, it could be sent up.

"Can I go to P.T. now? Twice a day, please? The sooner I start, the sooner you can throw me out of here."

"Heard from your father yet?" he asked as he wrote the orders.

How could *I* have heard anything? He had no idea where I was, while Dr. Hoffman was high on the list of people my father might call when he couldn't reach me. I had begun to sense an unspoken competitiveness among the potential callees, as if getting my father's hysterical phone call were some sort of prize, the winner receiving the "second most important person in my life" award.

I spent the entire morning in P.T., returning to my room for lunch, eager for my next session just hours away. By the end of the day, I was *standing* again! I knew the worst was over. This time, Dr. Hoffman was right.

"I *can* sit up in a chair, but the nurses wouldn't let me," I announced from my bed as he strolled in at the end of the day, reading Carol's notes in my chart. Was this the same person who had been so angry days before, so convinced she'd need a month to recuperate, so afraid even to sit up earlier the same day?

"I'll tell them you can do whatever you want."

"Great! And now you can tell my father some good news when he calls you in a state of panic." I was sure Dr. Hoffman would be the one to get the call.

As it turned out, my father had called the house. When there was no answer, he concluded I was out shopping. Of course, he started to worry, although I didn't *have* to be home, hours before his arrival in Mansfield. His connecting flight from New York City made a brief intermediate stop, and with anxiety overtaking reason, my father persuaded the stewardess to let him off the plane to place an urgent call. Still no answer. By this time he was alarmed but had no time to track me down. He spent the last twenty minutes of his long journey home in a total frenzy. Still, as I pointed out to him later, had I called him when I went to the hospital, his anxiety would only have been greater, and more protracted. Seconds after deplaning, my father was at the telephone dialing his home number once more. Still no answer. Now he had to make another call to find out where I was. Of course, he called my sister—his *other* daughter.

When the phone next to my bed rang, around 7:30 p.m., I knew who it would be. "Everything is okay. Would you mind stopping at Baskin & Robbins? The usual, please."

* * *

Friday, October 14: discharged! One week. It was hard to believe. What started out as a depressing setback turned out to be another blessing in disguise.

Because of my experience during the summer, I came to equate a compression fracture of the spine with a long, painful recovery—and abject dependence on other human beings for my most basic needs. Indeed, it was the dependence that made a compression fracture so much more serious than, say, a rib fracture, which I had suffered on several occasions. With a rib fracture, I had always been able to take care of myself and never lost even one day from work. The last week's ordeal taught me that a compression fracture need not be as devastating as I once thought.

I was also glad this episode occurred when it did, before I returned to work. It was better to laugh about fracturing my spine picking up a dead mouse, than to associate the accident with something important, like lifting a drawer from the card catalog in the library. The dead mouse story sounded silly, but also made me realize I hadn't *done* anything to cause the fractures. Clearly, these last two lumbar vertebrae were ready to go. If they hadn't collapsed from my picking up a mouse, they would have from doing something else. After fifteen years on steroids I was beginning to fully appreciate the meaning of "spontaneous" fractures. I was lucky my bones had lasted this long.

Leaving the hospital, for the *fourth* time in 1983; climbing into the sunken front seat of my father's Toronado; driving to the grocery store; strolling slowly through the aisles, my cane replaced by the shopping cart for support—I grew more and more amazed at how far I had come in the last week. And the last months. Arguing with my father over whether we couldn't buy some shrimp to celebrate—I would use any excuse for extravagant eating—I suddenly recognized that while I could never have gotten through this year without him, I had gotten through a pretty rough week on my own. My self-confidence, like my body, had become "porous" and weakened during the past year. At times I had wondered if it would ever return to its previous state of well being. When my father and grandmother departed for Israel, I thought this would be an opportunity to regain some of my lost self-confidence. Managing the house on my own, driving, doing a few hours of volunteer work, would have been enough of a boost. Handling the dead mouse incident more or less on my own was a much more significant accomplishment.

Eighteen

> Health alone does not suffice. To be happy, to become creative, man must always be strengthened by faith in the meaning of his own existence.
> —Stefan Zweig

One month after my discharge from Lyman Memorial I was ready for a trial run of living alone in my apartment. I hadn't told anyone at work I was coming to Concord, and didn't plan to visit the library. I didn't want to announce my plans too soon, in case I felt like chickening out at the last minute. Also, I wanted to be alone for a few days, to see just how much I could do. I knew that if my friends learned I was in town, I would quickly be over-booked with social engagements. It was a fun idea at first thought, but sure to be overly taxing.

Since most of my belongings were still in my apartment, I didn't need to bring much with me—a good thing, given that I couldn't, and wasn't supposed to, carry anything heavy. Carrying my own body around was more than enough. I spent most of the weekend in front of the television, knitting, reading, basking in the feeling of recovering—as if I were with my father in Thornden, but instead alone in Concord.

Actually, it was easier to function in my apartment than at my father's house. There was no staircase to climb, no soft sofa to sink into, no heavy glass shower door to pull and push, and the expanse of only a single room to traverse. My studio apartment, which in the past often seemed claustrophobically confining, now became a boon, everything I needed located within a small space.

I stayed in Concord only three days. It was long enough, with so little to occupy me. I'd forgotten how much my routine had changed. Gradually, I had established a reasonably satisfying schedule of activities in Thornden, balancing "work," exercise, and rest: going to the library to do volunteer work, continuing physical therapy on my own at home, cooking dinner most nights for my father. It was not so bad. I decided it was best to make several short trips to my apartment, each time staying in Concord a little longer, each time adding something new to the days' activities.

I returned to Thornden to find a thick envelope from the Social Security Administration waiting for me. I'd always associated thick envelopes with good news. Rejection letters were never longer than one page. I was right. Inside the envelope was my "Social Security Award Certificate," dated November 2, 1983. "Award Certificate"—what an odd name for it. I began to read through the package. "Type of Benefit: Disability. Date of Entitlement: July 1983. Monthly Benefit: $464.10." Now that I was almost ready to return to work, I was "certifiably" disabled. Enclosed with my Award Certificate was a pamphlet, "Your Social Security Rights and Responsibilities—Disability Benefits." One of the responsibilities listed was to inform the Social Security Administration of changes in my condition, especially as they pertained to my ability to work. I saw no reason to report my volunteer work. I preferred to define that as therapy, no different than "working" at home, writing book reviews for a leading library journal (which I had continued to do all year), or typing transcripts for my friend Kate, who needed help with her dissertation. I also saw no reason to inform the Social Security Administration of my intentions to return to work in January. For the time being, my (semi) permanent residence was still in Thornden, with my father. Although I grew increasingly optimistic about returning to my normal way of life, I had a superstitious fear that something *else* could still go wrong.

I drafted a letter to the Social Security Administration dated December 31, 1983, giving them my change of address along with my expected work schedule and salary, and filed it away. I looked at the award certificate one last time. It stated that I would receive another check for "back benefits," for the months from July through October, in the amount of $1,856. "Back" benefits. How appropriate. As I started to contemplate how to spend that windfall, I knew I was getting better, feeling like myself again: first, you buy!

* * *

During the next few weeks I caught up on the missed medical upkeep of my body, visiting my dentist, ophthalmologist, gynecologist, and Syd. I had originally planned my appointment with Syd as little more than a social call, there being no urgent need for me to see a dermatologist. But more than any of my other physicians, except Dr. Hoffman, Syd had seen me through this past year. He literally "held my hand." Sometimes he'd stop by my room at midnight, on his way home from the hospital. I owed him the pleasure of seeing me walk into his office on my own two feet. He had insisted all summer that I'd walk by Labor Day. We even bet on it. He was right. Again.

Meanwhile, however, my father had discovered a melanoma in the arch of his left foot! He'd noticed a tiny but alarming black spot while bathing in the Dead Sea. The day after he returned to Thornden, he had it removed. This gave Syd a fresh reason for giving me a real examination. If a person has a melanoma, his blood relatives are more likely than the norm to develop one too. Having survived so much, we were not about to let some suspicious-looking mole get out of control. Knowing Syd, I suspected he'd find at least one candidate for his knife. He found two: one for Blue Cross, one for Blue Shield.

Before returning to Concord, I wanted to tie up all the remaining loose ends I'd created during the year. My last day at the School of Nursing library, I "worked" longer than ever, four solid hours, the same schedule I planned to have at my real job come January.

Next, one last meeting with Carol, for a drink, not physical therapy. Finally, a special dinner at Yinky's with Dorothy. How things had changed since she had to hoist me into the shower, had to hold even a lightweight hair dryer for me, had to push me around in a wheelchair. More than anyone else from this year's cast of characters, I was happiest not to need her anymore, for she symbolized the worst of my helplessness. Yet, despite my association of her with such unpleasant events in my life, I had nothing but gratitude and good feelings for her.

*   *   *

Eva and Michael flew into town two days before Christmas. They were astonished when they saw me. They knew I was "better." But they also knew me as they had seen me last, six months earlier, barely recovered from the splenectomy and freshly disabled with compression fractures of the spine. With the thrill of seeing my remarkable improvement and our reunion behind us, we looked around the house and discovered that something was missing. There was no Christmas tree in the living room and less than forty-eight hours until Christmas! My father had long been determined to wean his children from this ritual, now that we were grown up. He had a whole list of objections, none having anything to do with his atheistic philosophy. It was a waste of money; it was a nuisance to haul it home and set up; and most of all it was a mess to clean up the thousands of needles scattered about the floor, and he would be left alone to dismantle and dispose of the tree. Still, this was not the year for him to start the new regime. I easily prevailed on his guilt, pleading that, after all, I should have been *dead* by now. Didn't I *deserve* a lousy little tree? This was not my first use of the "I should be dead by now" routine. Nor would it be my last. Why give it up as long as it works?

On occasions such as these, we naturally recall years past. Despite its joyousness, Christmas can also be sad and stressful. As we sat in the living room eating caviar and smoked salmon and drinking Piper Heidsick Brut, I thought about Christmases past, the good and the bad; about this cruel, seemingly endless year; about the uncertainty of the future. I thought back to 1968, when I first became ill, the last time I'd had such a rough time. Fifteen Christmases before, I had been too sick to go to school, too weak to help decorate the tree or help prepare dinner, and too frightened to enjoy the festivities. That Christmas was worse, much worse. I was going downhill then and there was no telling where my decline would end. This year, I had been through a similarly life-threatening crisis. But the worst was over. I was ready to go back to my apartment, back to work, back to *living* again with a chronic illness.

Epilogue

> The world breaks everyone and afterward many are strong at the broken places. But those that will not break it kills. It kills the very good and the very gentle and the very brave impartially. If you are none of these you can be sure it will kill you too but there will be no special hurry.
> —Ernest Hemingway

It was not easy to return to the library in January of 1984 after nearly a year's absence. I was fortunate to be working for people who were willing to hold my position open for me while I was sick and who let me return to work half time and increase my work load gradually. I appreciated their efforts and compassion, and I'm sure they knew it. But I also know that my dedication and hard work earned my employer's respect.

After I had been out sick for six months and placed on long-term disability, my supervisor was free to find someone to fill my job. Judith chose not to. She wanted me back as much as I wanted to be back. That was a burden on her and on everyone else in the Reference Department. It was also a tremendous encouragement for me to know I had such loyal friends and my job waiting for me.

When I returned, I continued to wear my corset during daytime hours, not only to support my back but also to keep me from inadvertently moving in a sudden and potentially dangerous fashion. I was afraid I might reinjure myself and become helpless again. This was a legitimate fear that I knew only time would diminish. In the meanwhile, I wouldn't let my anxiety show. I put on my best face to counteract my colleagues' concerns that I needed special treatment. *That* I didn't want.

* * *

It is now five years since I returned to work at the library after the longest absence and the most serious lupus flare I've had since the onset of my illness. It is ten years since I moved to Concord and became a professional librarian. And it is twenty years since I first became ill and was diagnosed with systemic lupus erythematosus. Milestones, all. Commemorating events in life gives me a sense of order. Even when I can't remember an exact date, I remember certain days—some good, some bad—that have made me the person I am today. I remember especially the day I fried myself on the beach at Cape Cod.

Something in the early years of my life must have prepared me to deal with the difficult times that followed, so abruptly, often so relentlessly. I remember relatively little of those early years, and nothing particularly unusual. I think I was like most of my friends: reasonably healthy, reasonably happy, comfortable, financially secure, and bright. These were all the ingredients for a promising future. I don't know where any of my eighth-grade classmates are today, what they have done with their lives, whether they are proud of their accomplishments and at peace with themselves. I know that I am—perhaps because just getting here turned out to be so much more difficult than I expected twenty years ago.

Today, I feel better about myself than ever. My lab work still shows lupus activity, I still have joint pains and a low-grade fever, and I must still take a moderately high dose of Prednisone (10 milligrams, twice a day) to keep my lupus under control. Although my lupus has been relatively quiescent these last five years, I still see Dr. Hoffman every two months. While this may be excessive, it gives us both a sense of continuity, more of a sense of control than we really have. By now, Dr. Hoffman trusts me, indeed expects me, to push myself, knowing I won't do anything foolish. That is not to say we always agree about which activities are foolish. He insists, for example, that I cannot ice skate because I might break my bones. But when I confessed to cracking a rib and simultaneously contracting a bladder infection while in the company of a not-so-young man who shall remain nameless, he was pleased to hear I was enjoying a "normal" life again. Employing this risk/benefit strategy, I tried to argue that skating was just as pleasurable. I got nowhere. I guess Dr. Hoffman is into watching basketball games.

I'm still convinced I'm not as pretty as Eva. But now I'm thinner than she is, and she is very slim. I wish I could say the same about being under-height: I am now *very* short, shorter than I've been all my adult life. The compression fractures of my spine cut three inches from my congenitally small stature. *I* find the difference noticeable, perhaps more than other people. At four-foot-ten, I thought of myself as petite. At four-foot-seven, I feel just plain *short*.

There are many things I love that I've had to give up in recent years, such as skating; and many things I've given up I can easily do without, such as walking a mile to and from work every day. Instead, I swim almost every day, usually as much as a mile. When Dr. Hoffman told me to give up skating and start swimming, I felt angry. I didn't want to give up something I enjoyed for something I considered merely therapy. Swimming may not improve my osteoporosis, but it might slow its progression. Weight-bearing exercise is better for maintaining bone mass. But my bone mass is so wasted it can't withstand that kind of stress. And while swimming may not help my bones much, it is certainly good for my muscles.

* * *

Why did I ever decide to work full time again? I don't need the extra money. What I need is the knowledge that I can do it. I am now a senior member of the staff, a specialist sought after to answer intricate reference questions, the assistant to the deputy director of one of the largest research libraries in the country.

Working full time, there aren't many hours left in the day, and I haven't been willing to decrease my social activities. To make sure I wouldn't miss an invitation to dinner or the movies, I recently added a telephone answering machine to the gadgetry in my apartment. When I return home at the end of the day, I look forward to the red light flashing, signalling a message.

One day I had two messages waiting. I assumed one would be, as usual, from my father. The second was unexpected.

BEEP. BEEP. "36,000 platelets. Call me."

I recognized the voice instantly, but I had to play the tape back a second time, and a third. It was Carol, my former physical therapist. We were good friends now, and had kept in touch the last five years. I had talked to her only a few weeks before.

"Carol? What's going on? 36,000 platelets?!"

"Susan, you're not going to believe this. I have thrombocytopenia! I just saw Dr. Jones. Remember him? He thinks I might have lupus, too. Maybe I should tell him I caught it from you, that it's contagious, with a five-year incubation period."

I could see why Carol and I got along so well, even when I had been in such terrible shape. We could always laugh at ourselves.

"Very funny, Carol. That's really terrible. What are you going to do? I suppose you know the options."

"I'm not sure. I think it's driving Dr. Jones nuts that I know you. Every time he describes some test or mentions a possible treatment, I interrupt him and say, 'I know about that from Susan.' I told him I want to have a splenectomy. But he wants me to go through a trial on Danazol, an anabolic steroid, first. I agreed. At least *I* won't turn to mush like you did on Prednisone."

"Maybe you should get a second opinion. Remember Dr. Ernst? He was much more favorably inclined toward splenectomy than anyone else, even for *me*. Why don't you go see him?"

"I thought of that. But Susan, you *really* won't believe this, either. He has been very ill . . . lymphoma, I've heard."

Carol didn't say so, but it sounded as though Dr. Ernst was dying. I was dumbstruck. Dr. Ernst was so full of life, a really lovable maniac. In the last few years, two of my favorite doctors had died: Dr. Patterson and Dr. Hauser. Was I about to outlive another?

"The secretary at the Hematology Clinic said Dr. Ernst is out on permanent sick leave," Carol continued. "I'm planning to see Dr. Cheever, whether Dr. Jones likes it or not. I know I'm going to end up having a splenectomy, and what better surgeon for the job. If he could fix you he could probably fix anyone!"

The news about Dr. Ernst put me in no mood for jokes. After a long telephone conversation listening to Carol's plight, I was stunned and exhausted. I got off the phone and poured myself a glass of Johnny Walker Black. I thought about Carol, and Dr. Patterson, and Dr. Hauser, and Dr. Ernst. And I thought about myself.